I0463989

One Man's Walk Into Medical Marijuana

An Experience by

Jeremiah Kush

Copyright © 2013 Jeremiah Kush

All rights reserved.

ISBN: 1481931253
ISBN-13: **978-1481931250**

FOR QUESTIONING MINDS

This book has to do with alternative medicines that may not meet some people's standards of morality. Maybe these people don't know the misery of sleep deprivation or have never felt the hammer of never ending pain. This is a story about how one man's suffering led him into a fast pace walk into legalized medical marijuana. The story tells of the surprises, the pitfalls, the plusses, the ease and the somewhat shady industry they call Legalized Medical Marijuana.

Chapter One: *The beginning*

Once upon a time in the shadowy darkness of Getting Old, I found myself sitting in my ever so familiar Lazy-Boy recliner pondering at sixty years of age, why it felt more like what I imagined ninety would feel like. In the last few years arthritis and other maladies have taken a costly toll on me and the way I was used to living my life. It all started about five years ago. Before then, my life was spent doing anything challenging, demanding, and most of all, it had to be exciting. This included football, surfing, scuba diving, snow skiing, and spending almost every summer backpacking in the great Sierra Nevada Mountains. I could get up in the morning at 7:00 AM and work on one of my five hobby cars until six at night; grab a quick shower and take my girl out to dinner and dancing. I could get up the next morning and do it all over again. Whatever happened to the good old days?

Five years ago I was finally getting around to remodeling my home when an irritating tingling in my fingertips started to bother me. The harder I worked, the stronger the tingle became. As time went on the tingle slowly started moving up both my arms. My hands were becoming numb all the time; work or no work, just a dead numbness. The only way I can really explain how it feels is something like this; imagine you put several pairs of those doctors' latex gloves on. When you touch something like a dime or rub your hand up the bare back of your spouse, you really can't feel anything; just that your hand is there and if you didn't have your eyes on what you were doing, you would have no idea what you were touching. On the other hand, though, if you took a hammer and slammed it down on the back of your hand, you would feel it in no uncertain terms. This is exactly how my hands feel. I can't feel a thing at skin level, but when I move my fingers, the pain of the arthritis comes through loud and clear. I can cut my hands or blister them with heat and never know it; but when I pick up a coffee cup, the pain hollers at me in a very loud voice. A voice I have become very tired of hearing.

Well, you know men. If they don't have a wife demanding they go see a doctor, nine out of ten times they won't. And I was, of course, one of those nine. For some reason, men think a problem will go away on its own; and nine out of ten times it won't. And yes, mine was one of those nine times it didn't go away; it slowly got worse over a period of years. What started out as a little tingle in my fingertips over time worked its way to my wrists; then, on up my forearms to the elbows, and now it's worked itself all the way up to my shoulders. When I sit around doing nothing my hands and arms are numb; you know, the latex glove feeling. That's not so bad. I can deal with that. The problem is when I over do the exertion to my hands and arms. Unfortunately, it doesn't take much to overdo it anymore. Now just a little work will make my arms tingle like I had slept on them wrong. More work will add a burning on top of the tingle; a burning somewhat like terrible sunburns; but a burn no lotion will soothe. The next level is the top of the terrible list. This is when it gets so bad I wouldn't care if the Doctor told me he would have to cut my head off; let's get on with it. Nothing can be as bad as this day in and day out. I'm not sure if my words can explain just how it feels, but just try to imagine licking both your index fingers and sticking them in an electrical wall socket. The burn and buzzing from fingertip to shoulders is relentless. It puts the numbness, the tingle, the sunburn and the stiffness to shame; and unfortunately, it usually continues until rest and no activity will bring it back to the old familiar 24 hour a day of just numb and tingling; a thousand times better than a wall socket sucking the life out of me.

So, off to the doctor I reluctantly decided to go. The man stuck me and shocked me; he X-rayed me and MRI'd me. Then, they sadly informed me the problem was caused by arthritis and calcium deposits in my neck vertebra pressing against my spinal cord; a type of spinal stenosis. Over time the growth started pressing on my spinal cord and the nerves leading out my spine and down to my hands. They tried intense therapy and several medications…neither of which did a darn thing accept empty my wallet. Since I was getting worse, not better, they decided I better go see a surgeon to find out if he could help me; his prognosis was nothing I wanted to hear.

According to the surgeon, the problem is in the fifth and sixth vertebrae of the neck; and the seventh and eighth don't look good. The procedure to surgically relieve the pressure is by going through the front of the neck near the Adams Apple and saw about a half an inch of vertebra away so they can remove that part of the spine from my body. At that point my neck will be held open and my spinal cord will be laying there exposed to God and country. They will then grind away at the inside of the vertebrae until the points of pressure will be removed. When that is completed to their very strict standards, they will reinstall the vertebrae; graft the removed bone with little pins, and WALA! No more numbness in my hands. You can't even begin to imagine how wonderful that sounds to a tormented man. But, no! Things never happen the way they're supposed to happen when I'm involved. And unfortunately, I'm totally involved right up to my numb and tingling neck.

I must say I was very disappointed when the Doctor didn't think the very complex surgical procedure would fix my particular problem; and that news, my friends, was about as welcoming as the plague. To make a long story short, the good Doctor tried to explain he felt, at this time, the procedure wouldn't help very much even if it went smoothly; which is nowhere near a sure thing. Losing the use of my arms and maybe even my legs is not out of the realm of possibilities and he made it abundantly clear. Being the big chicken I am the thought of an open spinal cord is not a good scenario to contemplate. The Doc's only advice was to continue therapy and the epidural shots I receive in the neck three or four times a year, which I must say, is now helping a lot.

Obviously there was not much I could do but watch the intensity of how hard I work very carefully. I have to make sure I don't overdue anything or I'd be paying for it later that night; a thought that scares the hell out of me. But no matter how smart I am, I can also be really dumb. You know, just a little more and I'll be finished, dumb. If I stop now I have to come back out tomorrow, so a little more won't hurt anything.

Stop, you idiot, stop! Why? Why should I stop now when I can get it done today; and yes, when I didn't listen to myself, I always paid for it later that night; a price never worth paying. But fear not, my friends. I have slowly learned to be smart, not dumb. After a few nights of howling at the moon, I've learned a hard lesson; and that hard lesson is now totally accepted in the deepest reaches of my gray ganglia. I can't do at sixty what I once did when I was twenty. But damn, I sure wish I could get to the point I could do more than just a lousy quarter of it. At this time in my life, if I could only do half as much as I did when I was twenty I'd be singing a happy song. Now, let's get on with the story.

One holiday season I was at a party with a bunch of old friends I hadn't seen in years. I happened to tell one of my friends, who will remain nameless, about my plight with numbness, tingling, and the dreaded wall socket. My life seemed to be in a downward spiral I couldn't control. Every little thing was becoming a major chore I found harder and harder to accomplish. I literally had to fight myself to do the simplest things; things most people, including myself a few years ago, would've considered simple everyday chores you don't give a second thought too. Things like the Post Office, grocery store and gas station seem so difficult to get myself to do; I mean a real battle. I would actually put off the grocery store until there wasn't a crumb in the house. The only thing I did was what I had to do; what was absolutely necessary to do. Other than that, whatever was usually put off until the "have to do" stage; and even then some have to do's, wasn't done. Everything I loved I hated; everything I hated I despised. I told my friend it was like walking around with my mind in a fuzz not being able to enjoy anything but a short nap; and a nap was about the only thing I looked forward too; an there's my problem. I constantly walk around in total and terrible fatigue. I told my friend I was exhausted all the time because I could never get a good night sleep. When I would fall off to sleep, it would never be more than an hour before I would wake up thinking my arm was asleep and I was laying on it wrong. I would usually sleep about an hour before I would wake. An hour or two later I'd fall back to peaceful sleep only to be awakened by the same nemesis sixty minutes later; and I'd be up at least an hour; usually two. I would fall back to sleep and a short hour later I would be awake like it was midday. This is how every night of my life was; and it was considered by me to be a miserable existence.

Now, of course, I told the Doctor about my little problem and he prescribed several sleep medicines, of which I won't give brand names because what doesn't work for me may well work for you; but the brands I took didn't seem much better than no sleep at all. With one I was so groggy when I woke, I couldn't think logically until ten in the morning. I didn't like that one at all. Even worse was the next one. It gave me the most horrible nightmares I've ever had; I mean the worst. One dream I was chasing my Dad with a butcher knife because he scratched my 1970 Hemi Barracuda. I woke up really wanting to kill him for scratching a car I never owned or even liked. This sounds funny now, but when I woke up in a pool of sweat and with a violent emotion I haven't felt since…ah, let's just say it was a time long ago and not worth remembering. Obviously, those sleeping tablets don't get along with my chemistry, so it was back to sleeping whenever I got the chance; and it was never more than an hour at a time. Try that one for awhile. No, on second thought don't wish this on your worst enemy.

Anyway, all parties end as this one did. On the way out, my nameless friend followed me to the car and pulled from his pocket an item that floated my memory back to an earlier and carefree time; a marijuana cigarette. Back in the late seventies and early eighties I guess I did my fair share of Weed consumption. I'm proud to say; or maybe I'm happy to say or even lucky to say; I never got involved with hard drugs. Ah, well…I take that back because it was a lie most people make. Hard drugs are heroin, cocaine, meth, LSD, ecstasy and a list I could go on and fill a page with. I thank God I never got involved with those hard drugs because I had my hands full of the other hard drugs; real hard drugs. Most people know them as tobacco and alcohol; others know them as death and destruction.

Back when I was a young boy it seemed more people smoked than didn't. I'm not sure it was a percentage fact, but everywhere you looked, people were smoking. Most of our fathers smoked as did everyone in the movies. The TV was flooded with Cowboy's having a relaxing smoke out on some scenic open range or some beautiful woman explaining how refreshing and clean her particular smoke was. To a kid, it really did make it look like the thing to do. Now we know the only smoke there was the smoke being blown up a fourteen year olds butt.

We just finished talking about the sweet addiction of smoking. Now, let's talk about the other quicker and even more destructive substance than tobacco; and that is alcohol. I think most everyone has been involved, or has known someone involved with the mess alcohol can, and does, produce in abundant quantities. I was lucky. My parents weren't drinkers in any way, shape or form. If I ever went home and there was a beer in the Frigidaire, I would be shocked. Most of the time it was there due to some kind of get together my parents was putting on. I'm not sure if it was my mother who didn't allow alcohol in the house, or if my father was adverse to it. I can't see my mother, or anyone else for that matter, telling my father what he could or couldn't do; on the other hand, I can't see my father disrespecting my mother's view's and wishes in any way. As I write this I have become curios myself. I think I may have to ask my Father next time we speak; maybe there is a story behind no alcohol in our home.

Now, back to the subject of marijuana and what I thought about it back in the day; I liked it. I thought it was so much better than alcohol. It didn't give you a hangover and even better, it didn't make you think you were ten feet tall and able to take on the United States Marine Corps single handed. I've seen alcohol and those other mind altering drugs turn good and respectable people into absolute morons, halfwits and assholes. I've seen peaceful parties turn into brawls because some ironman couldn't handle his liquor. It continually confirmed the thought anyone under the influence of anything was more of a disgrace and a sideshow than a party guy or good timer. I didn't want to become one of them or even be associated with one of them. I felt that way because I knew at a young age I had a particularly addictive personality. If I liked it, I would jump on it with both feet as I did with cigarettes, Scotch whiskey, marijuana back in the 70's, or even physical activities such as skiing, scuba, hiking, biking and restoring old cars. If I got into it, I got into it big.

Then, something happened with the occasional use of the marijuana part of the equation. It seemed technology found out how to measure it in your body; not if you're under the influence, but if you used it in the last week or two. They also started something called drug testing and random drug testing. Marijuana had become an enemy of society and I was smart enough never to battle society. I figured I'd lose every single time. Since there is no high on earth worth losing your job, livelihood and the ability to put food on the family table, I reluctantly gave the good old Doobie a found goodbye never to think about it again; that is until my nameless friend pulled one from his pocket on a clear cold New Year's night.

"Is that what I think it is?" I asked Nameless?

"Well, that depends on what you think it is," came the reply.

I knew damn good and well what it was. Back in the day we called them a "pinner"; a marijuana cigarette rolled to about one quarter the size of a regular cigarette. I held my palms toward him as if to say, "Not this week, my old and dear friend. I haven't messed with that shit since Reagan was in his first term." I then tried to explain smoking pot was not my bag and I was too old to partake in things illegal. I was far too old and smart to let myself get busted for driving home under the influence. He gave a chuckle and slipped it into my breast pocket.

"I see there are a few things you're not up to date on," he said with a smirk. Then my friend started to give me a brief explanation about the new marijuana; medical cannabis as he called it. To my surprised, Nameless had been a medical marijuana user for over a year. I had heard about medical marijuana, but that was all I knew about it; except I thought it was a scam of some sort or the other. Other than that, I never paid attention to medical marijuana in any way and never knew anyone who used cannabis for medication or even recreation reasons (that I knew of). I must say I was shocked to hear my friend used it to reduce the effects of his nausea. He told me it was the only thing that would keep his head out of the toilet and, to him, it was a God send. Since I was O-so-familiar with the marijuana munchies; you know, I could eat a box of Oreos and a quart of milk at three in the morning and when the cookies were gone, I contemplated eating the box. It sure seemed plausible a joint might rid you of nausea; maybe the Mithbuster's would even call it confirmed. But my problem wasn't nausea; it was pain, numbness and tingling. Getting so stoned you can't feel a thing is not my idea of pain management. Nameless simply laughed and said, "If you have to get rip roaring stoned for it to work...it's not working". He told me to take it home and give it a try when I was up against the wall and ready to take that long walk on a short pier. I shook his hand and wished him a Happy New Year. When I got home I actually felt a bit uncomfortable with a joint in my pocket. I considered giving it the flush, but I threw it in the junk box on top of the bureau instead; it sat there for months.

One morning I planned to change the radiator in my 1974 Datsun 260Z. It is a simple job with only four nuts and bolts and two radiator hose clamps holding it on. I started at seven in the morning and had the radiator off by eight. A job I would have knocked out in twenty minutes a few years back. After an hour in to Los Angeles and an hour back, I started to install the new piece. Four lousy bolts; only four lousy bolts I needed to mount the new aluminum radiator. When you can't see the bolt and have to reach down blind with numb hands to start a small eleven millimeter nut, you just can't imagine how many curse words fly every time you drop the S.O.B. and find your hurting body laying flat on your belly trying to find a simple little nut that so expertly camouflages itself on the black asphalt. After two hours of this total frustration, I sat on my butt, leaned against the car, and literally cried like a baby. Two lousy hours that once would have taken a few minutes. All my life I have depended on the used my hands for both work and play. When you take away a man's hands, you take away a big part of his existence. On that depressed moment of my life I was so deeply disappointed I literally felt my life had no meaning. What I used to do in a snap, I fought with everything I had just to complete the task. When you start to feel your life has no meaning, you better take serious note because nothing but bad can happen. I was exhausted and so very depressed I knew I had a very serious problem and it was time I better start worrying about myself; I felt useless and I saw no way out of the deep, dark dilemma.

Later that night, after the fiasco with my 260Z, I was paying the price I knew would be waiting for me. Earlier, as I was working, I knew I'd be hanging on to that lousy wall socket like there would be no way to pull from its evil grip; but on that night the buzzing was so extreme it seemed more like it was trying to kill me. I tried everything I knew including 800mg of ibuprofen and a very hot shower aimed right on the back of my neck. I already knew alcohol wasn't the answer; all I'd be was drunk with the same relentless buzzing; not to mention an almost as bad hangover the next morning. Believe it or not, a hot shower seemed to help more than anything. It took the buzzing in my arms and reduced the pain from the unmanageable nine down to a manageable five or six. While standing in the shower with the hot water on my neck and bubbling down my arms, I can't even feel the neck and arm problems what-so-ever. That's why I liked long and hot showers so much; and at the time, it was the only thing I knew to do…but wait. There's the doobie in the box on the bureau that's been sitting around for months. Do you think it's worth giving a try?

I must say I sat there for quite a while pondering the plus and minuses of lighting that baby up. But, man, at that moment I think I would have tried anything to get some relief.
So, into the bedroom I went with trepidation on what I was about to do; and to tell the truth, I thought I was about to turn myself into a criminal; or at least, something that is averse to being a solid

citizen. Benedict Arnold or not, there I went looking for the things I needed. Matches were the first on the list of things needed. But, geez, where do I find a match? I don't think I've seen one in years. You know, I think there might be a lighter in the Hotrod. Nope. Wait a minute. I know there is a lighter next to the propane torch in the garage. OK. Now I have the light, I now need the proverbial roach clip. Wow, I think I'm out of luck on that one. Maybe a pair of tweezers from my Swiss Army knife; but where the heck is that? Oh, well. I think I'll just smoke half. If I do, I won't be bothered with the need for a clip.

So, with great apprehension I put the illegal substance to my lips and lit that puppy up. After a fairly deep draw I was actually surprised I didn't cough or choke. After two or three more pulls on the tiny cigarette, it was about half done so I set it aside with what I thought, at the time, was no reaction to the weed. I went back to watching TV with more than a little guilt on what I just did after so many years. It wasn't more than five or ten minutes before I noticed the buzzing in my arm went from an eight or nine down to a four or five; the sunburn feeling was virtually gone. Not only that, I seemed very relaxed. Some may call it stoned, but after months of a constant tingle, it seemed I was more relaxed than stoned. The next advantage was even better. Usually I go to bed around ten. I would always wake up at midnight or before; I would go back to sleep around one just to wake up again around two. Once I went back to sleep around three, I knew I'd be awake at four. Back to sleep at five and awake to stay up and start my day at six. From then I would try to catch a nap whenever my body would say sleep; and that would never be more than a half hour at best. Without long and deep rim sleep, a person just can't function right. Believe me, I know. It had been a very long time since I had a good sleep; that is until the night I kissed a little doobie a few times.

I went to bed around ten as usual. I don't remember going to sleep but I know it was right away because I started to watch NOVA and I didn't remember a thing about it. But that's not near what was best. When I did wake, I looked at the clock through sleepy and blurry eyes to find it was three-thirty. Three-thirty! I couldn't believe I slept from ten to three-thirty. Not only was I extremely happy I slept a straight five and a half hours, I felt I could roll over and go right back to sleep; which I started to do when I noticed there was light out my bedroom window. At first I thought the neighbor turned all the outside lights on, but it was the sky that was light. I looked back at the clock and found the time was not three-thirty; it was a very beautiful and welcomed five-thirty. It had been a very long time since I was as happy as I was that morning. I laid there thinking about it for a minute or two when, low and behold, I fell asleep again. This time I slept till seven.

I must say that morning I got up whistling a happy tune. I felt refreshed like I finally got a good night's sleep after four long years of being enemies with the night. There was no grogginess or hangover type feeling what-so-ever. With years of crying from agony, on that morning I wanted to cry with happiness. It was the first time in years I looked forward to the day ahead and what I could do with it. Man, I can't tell you how good it felt to sleep the whole night long.

The next night I wanted to smoke the other half, but the better part of me thought I might wait and use it when I really need it. Since I didn't have any more of the stuff, that last half of the little doobie was a very prized material. So instead of a good night sleep, I tucked it away for use at a later date when it might be of more value. It was only a few days afterward a TV show on CNBC called *Marijuana* caught my attention. A show like that wouldn't have mattered a bit several days before. I wouldn't have even noticed the show; but now, not only did I notice, I watched with intense concentration. What the show was saying was very intriguing and almost unbelievable. They talked about medical co-ops and how big a business it had become. They talked to growers, sellers, patients and lawmen; all of which seemed to be cloudy and contradictory at every turn. One minute they tell you its absolutely legal in California and on the next minute they tell you the Feds can haul your ass away for a long time. Knowing nothing at all about medical cannabis, this seemed awfully weird. Can you use this stuff without fearing a trip to the hoosegow, or is it something to leave alone? After sixty some trips around the sun I have never heard the steel bars slam behind me and I can assure you I will never come close to wanting to. On that particular night I was in such a quandary it made me sure what was needed was a lot more research into the matter.

Chapter Two: *Becoming State Legal*

I thought about the CNBC show for some time with intense scrutiny and analysis. I wasn't at all sure if this was something I should mention to my doctor or just forget about the whole contradictory thing. A few nights later my question was answered for me. You got it. I helped a friend move and as sure as you're sitting there, the dreaded wall socket reached out and grabbed me. So, with some reason to think positive, I pulled out my last little bit of hope, in the form of a half smoked doobie, and smoked it with great expectations; and brother did it come through for me in spades. I didn't sleep quite as long as the first time; but sleeping to three and then on to five-thirty was more than I could wish for. And better yet, I could roll over and be back to sleep in minutes. I hated to admit it, but I was thinking this was just what I needed. It was time to look into this matter with a lot more gusto.

It was near the end of April when I decided to see about becoming a full-fledged medical marijuana patient; but how? Where do I start? I guess when you're in the computer age the question is simple; on the computer, of course. When I searched medical marijuana, I must say I was very surprised when a million web pages came up; and one advertized to find a doctor near you. With that lead I called an office near me and made an appointment with a doctor for the following Saturday. My instructions were to bring all information on my ailment and what my regular doctor was doing about it; medications, therapy, etc. I was also told to bring one hundred and fifty dollars. If I passed, they would keep the money; if not, I kept it. I was starting to wonder what this was all about.

I have to admit I was a little nervous when I left my house to see the doctor. The office was nearby off the 605 freeway in a large major bank building. With my epidural report and two sleeping medicine prescription in hand I entered the office on the top floor. It was a modern an expensive looking room with a receptionist near the front door; a rather large waiting room was at the far end and two private rooms on either side was the entirety of the office. The young woman gave me a stack of papers to fill out before I could see the doctor. The papers gave the pros and cons on cannabis and the legalities of medicating; such as it must be used as a medicine and not as a recreation device; you cannot sell it or give it to friends. It also tells you where you can or cannot medicate and it has about another hundred things you can or cannot do. It took the better part of an hour just to fill out the paperwork, but I completed it and was ready to give it back to the receptionist. After she went over almost everything again, which took another twenty minutes; I was finally ready and able to see the doctor.

When I walked into the office with the windows overlooking the 605 Freeway, a very cordial woman of around thirty-five was there to greet me with her hand held out. Maybe I shouldn't have guessed her age due to I'm so bad at it. To me women are thirty-five or they're in the category of daughters, granddaughters, mothers or grandmothers. I mean my guesses have been known to miss by a decade or more. If I missed the Doctor's age, I would say she was on the thirty-side; not on the forty-side. All I knew she was on the Doctor-side (I think). As she looked at my medical portfolio, I looked around the office. I would say it looked like any other doctor's office, except in this office there was not much there. I saw no paperwork on the desk, no bookshelves with medical journals; not even a phone on the desk. The office did have a few doctor type certificates on the wall and a gurney with bare vinyl cushions and a stethoscope coiled up on the end. I assumed it remained there because the doctor didn't have the stethoscope when she entered.

"So, Mr. Kush," she asked with a giggle, "what brings you to a medical cannabis Doctor?"

At the time I was totally unaware of my name being synonymous with some of the best cannabis known to man until she explained the Kush was an area in North India and Afghanistan producing many strains of the best Indica and hybrids in the industry. She apologized for the chuckle and again asked me for my story.

I would guess after about twenty minutes of telling her just what I told you, the Doctor commented on my spinal stenosis in, I must say, very articulated and savvy Doctor terms. I mean those four dollar works she was spouting were the exact same words my Pain Management Doctor had been telling me for years. She also talked about the sleeping medication and the chemistry involved and how they affect the body and mind. After listening to the woman, I personally don't think a person could talk that freely about a medical condition without years of medical study and experience. If she wasn't a doctor, she pulled one over on me. That said, the Doctor proudly announced I was a prime candidate for the use of medical marijuana;

and on that particular moment everything seemed surreal to me. Just a few days earlier I wanted to know about medical marijuana and now I'm a California State certified, card carrying, marijuana legal, sixty-two year old man. Wow!

Now that the Doctor verified my eligibility as a marijuana patient, she began explaining every aspect of the herb and how you can use it to medicate. I guess, like me, we all know about intake through smoking, but what I really didn't know was smoking is just one of many ways to ingest the substance known as THC. THC (**Tetrahydrocannabinol**), as explained by the good Doctor, is the main cannabinoid responsible for the psychoactive high. It's by no means the only cannabinoid, but it's the one most experts consider to be the primary one; although, the mixing of cannabinoids will give different affects on the mind and/or body; but more on that later.

Other than smoking, she told me vaporizing was the alternate and healthier way of inhaling the medication. By the way, everyone in this field always refers to you as the patient and the marijuana is always the medicine. Now, vaporizing was a method I never heard of. The way it works is you have a small unit that warms the herb to a certain temperature below the burning point. The THC is extracted and breathed in through a tube

with a mouthpiece or a plastic bag can be connected
to the unit so it fills with vapor that can be breathed
up to many hours from the time of vaporizing. I
personally like this system the best; although I had
to laugh at myself when I heard about it.

Back in the day a friend of mine would grow
some weed in his backyard from the seeds he got
from a previously bought lid. (A lid is a baggie of
pot the size of an ounce or twenty-eight grams).
Who knows what the sub-strain or even the main
stain was. It was pot to us and our aim was to
smoke it. We would go out in the back yard
greenhouse and pull the biggest fan or Sun leaves
off the plant and head to the oven. We had no idea
the high came from the THC; the THC came from
the Trichomes and most of the Trichs were located
on the bud, or flowers, of the female plant. I don't
think we knew what a bud was and I'm darn sure
we didn't even know marijuana plants came in male
and female varieties. Even though the female plant
is prized and the male plant and seeded female is
junk, it was all marijuana to us. With those fan
leaves in hand and the oven on a very warm 350
degrees, they were placed on a cookie sheet and
popped into the oven with us being totally unaware
THC will start to vaporize around 190 degrees. We
were using the worst part of the plant and burning
off most of the THC, to boot. And if I remember

right, we sat around listening to the Doors or Joe
Walsh thinking it was pretty good shit. Boy, if we
knew then what I know now.

OK, now we've talked a little about smoking
and vaporizing. The next way of ingestion is by
way of eating. Now, you just can't grab a handful
of weed and chow down on it like you're some kind
of herbivore; it will do you no good. The only way
to pull THC from the Trichomes is by way of fat or
alcohol, and of course, by way of smoking or
vaporizing. When eating it usually comes by way
of butter, a very fat heavy substance perfect for
drawing out most of the cannabinol. Just to give
you a little idea how it works is something like this.
You take some ground up bud and let it steep and
simmer in melted butter for a few hours before you
strain the muddle with a bit of cheesecloth. The
green substance is butter with a very earthy taste
and saturated with very strong medical THC. You
can use the concoction in any recipe just as you
would use normal butter; but your butter has a much
bigger kick. You can also cover a number of buds
in a jar with IPA, or rubbing alcohol, for several
days until the liquid is a golden color. The 90%
IPA works much better than the common 70%.
Shake often to help release the medication. You
then strain the liquid in a bowl and cover with
cheesecloth until the alcohol evaporates. Be sure to

do this in a well ventilated room with no source of fire. Remember alcohol is extremely flammable and should be treated with the utmost respect. When the alcohol evaporates you will be left with sticky oil looking a lot like honey or motor oil. You can utilize this very strong mixture by soaking some herb and smoking it the normal way, or you can saturate a cigarette paper when you roll a joint or smoke a Marlboro. The medication will come at you with much more gumption.

The last way is by drinking a tincture made with cannabis. This process is almost like the IPA alcohol, but you use a drinkable and very strong vodka, gin or rum. I'm talking one hundred proof or more. You let the trichome-heavy buds lay around in the booze bottle for a couple of weeks and you will have yourself a very strong martini that can easily put you three sheets to the wind. To me, mixing strong alcohol and strong marijuana seems like a little overkill. Walking around in a stoned and drunken stupor seems to me you're a very sick person or you're contending to be the Stoner of the Year. I'm not sure the latter is an award anyone would be proud to claim.

I'm told there are THC pills coming to the market and I've even heard they are working on an injection form of marijuana. Since I have absolutely no experience with any of this I can only say check the internet if you're interested.

Now, after the Doctor's explanations had been gone over and all of my questions answered, she had the receptionist make out all the paperwork. I had a medical card to keep in my wallet; a card to keep in my glove box and a card to keep at home. It was all neatly placed in a very professional folder and all was complete except for the exchange of the one hundred and fifty bucks for a year; renewals will cost a Ben Franklin. I then received a list of cannabis dispensaries in the area, and to my surprise, at that very moment I was able to go to any Co-Op dispensary and pick up the medication of my choice. I was very astonished on how fast the whole process took to complete. I said my thank you and walked out of the office a legal and certified medical marijuana patient for the next twelve months. Their last words to me were "see you in a year for your renewal. It's only a hundred bucks then."

Chapter Three: *The Co-Op*

Walking away from the doctor's office I wasn't sure if I was happy, excited, confused or just plain overwhelmed with what took place. I sat in the car to ponder what the next step should be because I felt I was so far in front of the curve. I wasn't sure if I was ready for the next step in the process; that be going to a Co-Op to pick up my medicine. And except for smoking it, there was really nothing left to do. Since there was a dispensary only a couple of miles from where I was, I decided I would go over and take a look and possibly buy something if I had the nerve.

Now I'm not exactly sure what I expected as the car made its way to a spot I never thought I'd be heading for. For some reason I thought a State authorized medical marijuana dispensary would be something like a CVS or Walgreens with pharmacy type folks in white jackets dispensing the weed; I couldn't have been more wrong.

I must have driven past the dispensary four times before I found it; and even then I wasn't too sure. The address brought me into your average type strip mall with everything from a 7-eleven to a carpet store. So, right between a Mexican bakery and mattress store was a narrow storefront of about fifteen feet wide. On the painted out windows was a small sign with the name I was looking for. The store front reminded me of one of those back in the day adult book stores peddling in pornography; you know, the plain and simple storefront meant to bring no attention. I almost kept driving, but my curiosity got the best of me. After parking the car and spending a few moments looking around the neighborhood for possible police, I was shocked at myself for thinking I was a criminal ready to go see my dealer. I watched several people walk out nonchalantly with a small bag in their hand, throw it in the trunk, and drive off like they just went into the 7-Eleven and bought a soda. All of them seemed to be in their twenties, which didn't seem quite right to me.

After a deep breath, I talked myself into going in. With heavy curiosity, I opened the door to find a small and very plain lobby with cheap tables and chairs at the far end. A few steps from the door were poles and ropes, kinda like the ones you would find in a bank, leading to a glass window resembling a movie theater ticket window. Behind the window was a young and very pretty girl. She couldn't have been much older than twenty.

"Have you been here before?" she asked as it seemed to me I was being studied thoroughly. I wasn't sure if I was out of the age bracket she was used to, or if I was just being self conscious and feeling a little out of the time. After I told her this was a whole new experience to me, she seemed to warm up as she handed me a pile of paperwork every bit as large as the one in the Doctor's office; and I would say the questions were identical. In return, I handed her the package the doctor gave me and, of course, my driver's license.

After returning the completed paperwork, she gave me back my driver's license and a new store identification card. She explained from then on out all I had to bring was my driver's license and their store card. They weren't interested in my personal medical marijuana card given by the doctor. The California certified card was just to get me through the door for the first time. From then on out, as she told me, I was a member of their cannabis club. She directed me to the door at the far end of the room and told me to wait until she buzzed me in. After a few moments the door opened as promised and I walked into a short hall with another locked door at the other end. Between me and the other door was an armed guard with a hand held metal detector. "Hello, Mr. Kush," came a happy greeting as he started to scan me with the hand held, "welcome to the club." Just then the buzzer on the hand held went off as he scanned over my pants pocket. He tapped the hand held on my pocket and asked, "Car keys?" When I told him yes, he explained there were never to be any kind of weapon brought into the club. This included guns, knives, brass knuckles, black jacks or any other thing they would consider a weapon. It was the only time the scanner was used on me.

When I agreed to all his rules, he opened the door and I followed him in. My first impression of the place was something or somewhere between a nineteen-eighty discotheque and a nineteen-sixty head shop. I took a quick second to look around the place. It was as narrow as the front and only twenty feet deep. I believe there is a storeroom or office in the back, but that's only a guess. The end of the room closest to the door found an overstuffed couch with a coffee table and a number of magazines; mostly *High Times*. On the wall in front of the couch was a large flat screen TV playing a DVD of their various strains of medicine and the medicinal qualities of each. At the other end of the room was a large glass cabinet of jars filled with different types of cannabis; all filled with nothing but buds. At the other end of the cabinet was everything imaginable when it comes to medicating. There were water pipes, bongs, rolling papers, screens, vaporizers, and things I had no clue about. On the wall behind the counter were items that looked like food items such as brownies, cookies and candies. There were also about a dozen marijuana plants about six inches high growing under the light. Before I could finish sizing up the place, I was pulled from my inspection by a cheerful voice. "Welcome to the club, Mr. Kush. How can I be of service?"

The kid reminded me of Richard Dreyfus in *American Graffiti.* I swear to God he could have been his younger brother. I began to explain this was an all new experience for me and I really didn't have a clue about any of it. As if he had heard it all before, he smiled and led me to the glass counter and introduced me to what they called the Budtender. I'm not sure if I can really describe this guy, but let me give it a try. First and foremost I want to start by saying the young man was very pleasant and even more helpful; but as I said earlier, I was expecting a Walgreens and white coats; not a tall drink of water with a six inch spiked Mohawk going from front to back; bright red in color. He wore leather jewelry with silver spikes around his wrist and neck looking somewhat like one of those bulldogs in a Bugs Bunny cartoon. The T-shirt he wore was black and silver with an Ozzie Osborne motif. Of course his denim trousers were as black as his Harley Davison motorcycle boots and both were adorned with silver chains; far, far from the pharmacy type I was expecting. But as I said, the kid was very nice and even more knowledgeable.

When I glanced at the board of items provided, the kid knew immediately I was totally confused. Walking in I thought I was going in to buy a baggie of marijuana, but I had no idea I would be looking at a menu closely resembling that of a Coney Island hot dog stand. I mean, you have your Sativa; you have your Indica, you have your hybrid; you have your edibles; and you even have your drinkables; and under those headings, you had several sub-strains like Purple Wreck, Dutch cheese, OG Kush, Blueberry Skunk, AK 47, Bob Marley's Sharks Breath, Peacemaker, Blue Dream, White Widow and probably a dozen other varieties. I had no clue to what I was looking at and I'm positive the kid knew it in an instant. When I shook my head he started explaining the various strains. First there is the Sativa plant which grows anywhere from five feet to almost twenty-five feet. It is prevalent in the equator countries like Columbia,

Thailand, Mexico and the Caribbean. The plant grows similar to a Christmas tree with a broad base and a single stem at top. The leaves are long and thin with a pale to medium green and a fragrance that's sweet and spicy. The plant is usually slow growing with a ten to fifteen week flowering cycle. The high can be anything from uplifting and social to psychedelic or mild paranoia. It really depends on your chemistry and how it affects you. Basically it is used more for the day and outside activities; so says the Budtender.

Indica's, on the other hand, comes from higher and colder regions such as the North of India and Afghanistan. Because of the different temperatures, the Indica plant is somewhat different from the Sativa. The Indica plant grows to only six feet at most with the base usually wider than it is tall. Its leaves are short, broad and deep-green with a pungent, sticky and fruitful odor to it. It grows more like a bush than a tree with a six to nine week flowering cycle. The Indica high is far more desensitizing and potent than that of the Sativa. Basically, Indica is used more for sleep and indoors; so says the Budtender.

Now, as I looked at the menu, I noticed several prices. They were all identified as "donation". When I looked at a strain called Northern Lights, the donation was listed at one hundred dollars. Now, when I bought Pot back in the day, it was ten dollars for a four finger bag, or about an ounce of weed. If you wanted the good stuff, you had to buy the Columbian for thirty dollars a bag. I was dumfounded the price went to one hundred dollars an ounce, and I told the Budtender I thought the price of one hundred dollars was a little high for a product that grows like a weed. The guy tried to control his laughing when he explained there was no price. Everything was a donation to the club. I don't think he thought it was too funny when I said, "If you don't have prices and only donations can the donation price be negotiated to half the going price per ounce?

Again, after the guy controlled his laughing, he simply explained this was no longer the seventies. And what he was about to say literally made my knees go weak. He informed me, with no regret or emotion, the donation of one hundred bucks did not get you the four finger ounce; it got you a measly one quarter of an ounce or seven grams if you prefer! In other words, he wanted me to pay one hundred hard earned dollars for a paltry equivalent of seven lousy cigarettes. He wanted me to receive the amount of seven cigarettes by weight for a one hundred dollar bill? Is this guy crazy? I mean after all, a quarter of an ounce is the same weight as those little candies about the size of an aspirin tablet. You know the ones. They're about two and a half inches long wrapped in clear plastic and twisted on both ends; well, my friends, that's a quarter of an ounce and one hundred dollars for such a small quantity seems outrageous.

I didn't even know if I wanted to hear anymore. I must have been flush with shock when the Budtender patted me on the shoulder and started to explain. "Sir, since this is no longer the seventies in marijuana prices, this is no longer the seventies when it comes to the potency of the cannabis, either. What you got in the seventies with a few doobies will now do the same with a puff or two. The groups in Amsterdam and other places have bred ultra high potency in the new strains of plants and they are getting stronger every day."

I wasn't sure about the potency he was talking about; all I wanted was a bag of the same stuff Nameless gave me and I sure didn't want to pay four hundred dollars an ounce to get it. I was still numb in regards to the price given me and I was searching for a way to get out of there, and I mean get out of there fast; but then, I started thinking about it. According to weedmaps.com there were several places in town that supplied marijuana. Should I leave and go through all the rigmarole of paperwork to find if another place was cheaper? The more I thought about it the more I realized the places were probably as competitive as any other establishment in the city. I decided to dig a little deeper before I checkout another Co-Op.

On the counter were little jars with red, blue and green caps; the red Sativa, the blue Indica and the green was the hybrid; a mixture of both Sativa and Indica. The jars were there with a bud or so for the patients to examine and smell each fragrance; which I must say I was shocked at the extreme differences in aroma. It went from fruity and floral to a pungent earthy skunk smell. I was starting to wonder what the differences were; if any. To hear the Budtender tell it, there are great differences; as different in the high as different in the smell. He explained since I wasn't a regular at medicating, I better be careful until I get use to potent medicine. For some reason that didn't seem to disconcerting to me at the time so I asked him what he recommended. Since I was new to the game he thought a middle of the road strength Sativa and a middle strength to a lesser strength Indica would probably be best. His choices were a Sativa called Sharks Breath and an Indica/Sativa mix called Sweet Tooth. He told me my response to the Sharks Breath Sativa would be an active, functional, social and talkative high; one for the daytime or outdoor use; whatever that meant. Sweet Tooth Indica was to bring about a long lasting and relaxing high to promote my much needed sleep. Boy did that sound good at the time.

Since I didn't want to put a marijuana dispensary on my Master Card, I peeked into my wallet for cash. I had one hundred and fifty dollars and a quarter of an ounce was a cool two-thirds of what I had. Since I didn't have enough to purchase a quarter of both, I thought I better go ahead and buy, I mean donate, the Sweet Tooth. I needed sleep more than I needed a talkative high to be use outdoors; whatever that meant. The Budtender then explained I could get it an eighth of an ounce if I wanted; I could even buy a gram if I wanted too. The price was like a lot of other things. The more you buy the better the price. So if you bought an eighth the donation was fifty-five dollars; a quarter was one hundred dollars and the once was a cheap three hundred and seventy five dollars; what a deal. What was even worse, some of the strains went for as much as one hundred and forty dollars for a quarter of a once or, seven grams if you prefer. The dispensaries always talk in grams and they won't sell you more than an ounce at a time. They keep your visits down to only three times a day and I couldn't help wondering who would go there more than once a month, much less three times a day. Again, I was having a hard time realizing I was standing in a room with countless jars of the best weed going and it was there for me as much as three times a day. I'm not sure that made sense to me then or now, but the thought of unlimited marijuana at my fingertips seem surreal or even totally unbelievable.

Well, it was time to buy the medicine and complete this unusual odyssey, so, I told the Budtender an eight of each and I watched him go to work. He took two full jars from the back wall and set them in front of me; Sweet Tooth as the Indica and a hybrid of Bob Marley's Lambs Breath and a strain called Great White Shark, now called Sharks Breath. I couldn't help but wonder who gives the title to all these strains and why they pick such weird names. I mean, I can understand Maui Wowie, Acapulco Gold and Sharks Breath; but Platinum Girl Scout Cookie, Sour Diesel and White Fire? The names sounded funny to me then as they still do now. As I thought about it he took a set of chop sticks from a jar filled with coffee beans. By the way, the beans were there so the patient could clear his or her palate with a big sniff so they could get a better fragrance between strains. Who would of thunk? I've learned since then to a lot of people this is right in line with wine tasting and all the superlatives that go with it. He then took the buds, one at a time with the cop sticks, and laid them on a digital scale. When the mark hit three and a half grams, he poured the buds in a little green plastic container with a lid that snapped closed. Of course, it had a label with all the legal ease stating this was for medical use only and was in ordinance with California State law proposition 215 and Senate Bill 420. It is not to be use while operating a motor vehicle and it is to be kept out of the reach of children and may cause drowsiness bla, bla, bla. Since I was a new customer I received a little glass pipe and two pre-rolled joints. And since it was free gram Saturday, you got a free gram with every quarter. That meant I got eight grams for the price of seven. Not too bad. The pipe was priced at six dollars; the joints were five dollars each and the free gram was about three and a half dollars; a savings of almost twenty dollars. Again, not too bad considering the whole of the transaction. But remember, I just spent one hundred and five dollars on the equivalent of a half pack of cigarettes. I never thought a weed could go for so much, and what's more, I never thought I'd ever even consider paying such a ridiculous price; but there I was digging deep into my wallet.

I handed the bills to the Budtender and he handed me a small brown bag stapled closed with the same label as on the jars. "Thanks for your business," he said with a smile as I took a bag of what I spent my life thinking was an illegal and somewhat useless substance. The way I was feeling, I almost felt scared to walk out of the place. Only a few short hours earlier I was getting ready to go see a doctor to see what she had to say on the matter. I never even thought I be holding a bag of Pot on the same day. I tried to explain my feelings to a kid whose life was as comfortable with cannabis as a kid in the 7-Eleven selling me a pack of smokes. I told him I was from the time a police officer would pull you over and tear you car totally apart and then leave all your seats, spare tire and anything else in your car all over somebody's yard or parkway. He was looking for what I was going to walk out with in full view; and that was eight grams of marijuana and all the paraphernalia to use it. I was way out of my comfort zone and I made the kid aware I was a little nervous about walking out and driving away.

Like it was no big deal at all, he just laughed and told me to put the bag in the trunk and drive straight home. If I follow all the rules there will be no problem at all. He said the taco stand a few doors down always pulls in the Sherriff for breakfast, lunch and dinner. Since it was lunchtime, I'm telling you, I almost fainted on that statement. But he continued on and told me in the two years he worked there only one of his patient's got stopped and that was due to an expired license plate and nothing to do with the medical cannabis. I have to say that made me feel a lot better, so I grabbed the bag of society's ill repute, said my thank you, and left more unbelieving than when I first drove up. I wanted to be as discrete as possible while walking out.

Chapter four: *Thinking About It*

Even with the Budtender's reassuring words I was still feeling very uncomfortable when I walked out of the place; and when I saw a cop car backed up to the taco stand, I felt even more uncomfortable. And of course, instead of having everything ready and organized for a seamless entry into the car, I looked more like a silent movie comedy star fighting every Murphy's Law snafu there could be before accomplishing the task. Since both my hands were full and I didn't want to put a bag of Pot on the roof when I got the car keys out of my pocket, I kept the Pot hidden and put the file with my medical marijuana cards up there instead. And sure enough, here comes a big gust of wind blowing the pamphlet and cards all over the parking lot. There I went, running all around like a chicken with its head cut off stomping on one card at a time trying to keep them from blowing closer to

the policeman having his lunch. OK, now I get all
the cards together and head back to the truck
wondering if the cop thinks I'm under the influence.
I didn't help the matter by dropping the keys on the
ground when I tried to slip them into the door lock.
Finally I got the truck door open, but it was just
that; a truck. It doesn't have a trunk. Now what?
The Budtender told me it was against the law to
keep it in the driver's compartment but what else
can I do? This thing only has a cab. (Note to self:
don't bring the Ranchero when you buy pot) Am I
supposed to throw it in the bed and let it bang
around or possibly even bounce out? Note at one
hundred dollars for seven lousy grams I'm not.
Geez, I got kinda brave when money came into the
question. Even a cop won't scare me when it comes
to letting a hundred dollar bill blow away. So
anyway, after thinking a minute, I decided to stuff
the bag into the little storage compartment behind
the seat. Since I figured the cop was staring right at
me, I made putting it behind the seat as obvious as I
could.

That done, I settled in and in another
obvious move I connected the seat belt and jammed
the key into the lock. Low and behold when I
turned the key I heard a sickening click, click, click.
Oh, man! That damned old battery cable again.
I've wanted to replace that thing for months now, so

why didn't I just get it done. With a deep sigh of disgust I pop the hood, undid the safety belt and walked to the front of the car. I could almost read the policeman's mind thinking I was here buying Pot and I couldn't even afford keeping my thirty year old driver running. I wiggled the cable and went back to give it a try. Thankfully the grey ghost started right up so I quickly closed the hood, redid the belt and put her in reverse. Oh, no, wait a minute. I don't have a front license plate. Here in California you need one. I've owned this truck thirty years and it never has had a front license plate. It didn't have one when I got the 78 Ranchero and now, of all times, is not the time I want to get pulled over for it. Maybe if I back out and go the other way he won't see it. Let's give it a try.

Well, as you guessed, the minute I drove away he started his patrol car and followed me; and yes, I thought my heart was going to bang right out of my chest. I'm not sure what it was, but even though I had everything I was suppose to have to make this thing legal, I couldn't help feeling like John Dillinger right after he heisted a bank. I nervously waited for the cars to clear before I turned right onto the boulevard with him right on my bumper. I proceeded to the first light and turned right; oh, man, he followed. This stretch of the road is a long way till the next signal and Mr. Copper followed me closely all the agonizing way. Just as I was pulling to a stop at the intersection, that sucker popped on the lights and gave me a heart attack at the same time. All I wanted was some relief from this numbness and now I'm going to have a full fledge coronary. Hell, now I won't have to worry about the numbness in my arms. The cures have killed me; but wait! He's pulling up on my right-hand side. Maybe he doesn't want me.

When the guy stopped at the crosswalk to check traffic, my window was down so he yelled, "Nice Ranch-a-roo. I had one just like it back in the day." He then clicked on the siren and took off like he was going to a murder in progress. Oh, man, did it feel like a ton of bricks were lifted off my diaphragm; I could breathe again. Now, I knew I could drive home with a lot more confidence and I did just that. Up to then, it was a very strange day and I was looking forward to getting back to normal.

I'm not sure when I got home anything was close to normal. I guess I have to say I was truly excited when I carried my new found booty into my bedroom and placed it proudly on the computer cabinet. I was giggling as I thought to myself what my family and friends would think when I tell them I'm a card carrying medical marijuana patient.

After setting out in neat little order the two jars of medicine, a little glass pipe, two joints, rolling papers, screens and a Bic disposable lighter, everything was ready to go; but wait a minute. Wait one cotton picking minute. When I saw all the Pot paraphernalia spread out in my own home it was like somebody gave me a hard slugged to the back of the head. It was like it told me to slow this horse down and think about what just happened. I mean, this happened so fast I really haven't given it very much if any thought at all. As I studied the items that only a few days ago I would have considered to be owned by a loser, I had to ask myself the hard question as to why they were in my home. Have I become a loser; will it drive me to become a loser?

That was a very scary thought so I leaned back in my chair and thought about it. I thought about it for a long time and I tried to cover every aspect I could before I went any further into this unknown venture. I even thought about driving home with the police on my ass. Since I was in my twenties I have had nothing but bad to say about the exact thing that was sitting in front of me. Man, this day has really wound up different than I ever expected.

I had to laugh at myself when I thought about it. I went from more paranoid than I have

ever been to more flattered than I'd ever been. I
was proud when the officer complimented my
Ranchero. I have always loved old cars and I can
prove it by owning a 1950 Pontiac, a1973 AMC
hotrod with flames, a 1974 Datsun 260Z, a 1978
FJ60 Toyota Land Cruiser and of course, the 1978
Ford Ranchero. All are restored and some done
several times. But no matter how much I love
working on cars and having people coming up to
me in a gas stations to admire my work, or
remember when they had one just like it; it brings a
pride on what I accomplished with five old rust
buckets. The problem with this scenario is old cars
constantly need work and work is what I can't give
them anymore. No matter how much it hurts to say,
it's the truth.

Anyway, that got me thinking even deeper.
With my Ranchero going to turn over a million
miles in the next two thousand miles, I had been
thinking very seriously about buying a brand new
car; you know, the kind that gives a ten year
warranty. It's exactly what I need; a reliable car I
won't have to worry about or wonder how I will be
able to work on it. And that's the rub. That was the
first time I really thought about the price of
everything and how much that everything went up
over the years. A quarter of an ounce didn't seem
like a lot of anything to me and at a hundred bucks I

wondered how long it would last. Obviously at about the equal of five or six cigarettes and you smoked a half of cigarette per medication you will get ten or twelve medications per quarter ounce jar. Wow, that works out to be around three hundred dollars a month. If you smoke more or better quality medication the price of marijuana is starting to push the price of a new car payment. I was beginning to be…not so sure about this little endeavor.

I also thought about the loser part, not just the removing of three hundred bucks plus from my monthly budget, and brother, that wasn't at all consoling and a big factor in my contemplation. But by now money wasn't all of it. As you walk through life, everyone comes across stories of how drugs and alcohol totally and mercilessly messed up a person's or even an entire family's life. I know it from a hard experience. My second wife became my second ex-wife because she wouldn't stop guzzling the booze. It eventually ended up killing her at a young age of fifty-eight. Since I divorced her at the age of thirty-six, you might say it was a long time to be stuck in a bottle and having a vicious monkey chewing on you back. At one time in my life I thought I would have danced on the table at the hearing of her death, but after twenty-three years I guess the hate and the pain of a broken heart mellows and softens over time. I guess it was the part of my heart that loved her once who commanded me to truly grieve for her. I know she was a much tormented woman for most of her life and I wish her peace and comfort in the Forever After. Pocks on abusing alcohol! The question is: is there such a thing as abusing medicine? Any idiot knows the answer is, "there sure as hell is."

But what about me? Do I have to worry about throwing everything aside for medical marijuana? Will this be any different than taking codeine for tooth pain, or stronger drugs for my once chronic back pains? Will this turn into a vicious monkey chewing on my back? I thought hard because I'll admit it to anyone; I've had my share of battles with the monkey and I have no enthusiasm to battle that son-of-a-bitch again. He's a hard fight and I'm not sure I have the power of youth, confidence and plans made far into the future to battle him again. I remember sitting there all alone in a melancholy mood remembering those hard fought battles kicking the irritating monkey off my own back. I didn't stop my mind from going back to an earlier day.

I was a young man getting ready for my senior year on the high school football team. Back then most "cool" people smoked including our fathers and grandfathers. Even though most people smoked, about the only thing people really thought about was it was bad for your wind. Most guys quit when hell-week started and most gave it up through the entire season. Now, at that time a young cocky fullback didn't believe in any such think called addiction. It was nonsense and if you wanted to quit smoking; quit. If you want to lose weight; quit eating. It's no big deal. And if you want to quit drinking, same old deal; just quit putting it to you lips. Boy, it sure was nice to be young and dumb.

So, back to the story. It was the end of summer and football practice was to start Monday. Being the last weekend of freedom we hit the beach, Knots Berry Farm and the local drive-in theater; and of course, we were smoking like chimneys and thinking we were big men in the adult world of automobiles, girls, cigarettes, and occasionally, a beer or two. So, Saturday night I was driving a group home after the movie and decided to have one last cigarette before practice started. I lit up a Pall Mall, looked at the three quarter full pack, and tossed them out the window. With the thought of no more cigs until after the season, I had no idea at the time I'd be wishing I never threw the pack of smokes away; and I really didn't even smoke that much. I'll bet a pack lasted me two weeks if not more. But if you have a smoke once a day, its way different than telling yourself they are a banned out of your life for months. If I remember right, it was pretty darned hard to get through the first month of school. I'm not sure why I didn't get the very direct hint from having a craving gnawing at me for an entire month. There I was, wanting a cigarette more than anything, but I banned them from use until after the season. It was so hard for the first month I always had to battle myself when I went to a store and saw them on the counter. But, by the time the season ended, I guess I forgot the temptation of those little boxes on the counter and what the monkey's teeth were like; or I was arrogant enough to think I could conquer and defeat any addiction enemy with little more than "just do it". And with that mantra on my mind and a minute after the last game of the season, there I was at the 7-Eleven for a pack of Camel lights. Come on boys; let's live life to the fullest! We're genuine bad asses!

We were just that alright. But now I know it was more ass than bad. And since wind wasn't required in golf, I didn't put a demand on myself for quitting smoking for another four years when I found myself in the workplace trying to support a family. But this time it was far harder than anything I ever experienced before. And when I say hard, for me it was by far and away the most miserable and difficult thing I ever did. I mean, I would walk around in a haze with this monster craving eating at me. It seemed like my skin would crawl across my body and since there was no smoke to dead my smell, food smelled and tasted better than I ever remembered. And since I was so on edge, there were things that caught my attention more so than usual. I remember one time I was in the employee cafeteria enjoying the same chicken soup I had been smelling and dreaming about all morning. At the same table was the security manager and a woman form accounting. When the woman asked why he wasn't drinking his morning coffee, he told her they just raised the price of coffee to 25 cents; which he thought the price ridiculous and he wouldn't pay it. (Good thing he didn't see the price of today's Pot). Anyway, the woman reached out and slammed a dollar bill on the table and told the man it was his. He reiterated her intentions of giving him the bill and when she confirmed she was giving him the dollar with no strings attached he pulled out a pack of cigarettes with a big wad of money rubber banded to it. He took the wad of money, rolled up the woman's dollar around it, wrapped it back with the rubber band and then he nonchalantly lit up a cigarette paying the shocked woman no mind. The woman wanted her dollar back; which she didn't get, and I wanted a cigarette because, boy did that cigarette smell good. But like the woman, no dollar for her and no cigarette for me. Even though it was as hard as anything I've ever done, I quit for six long years and told myself I'd never go through that hell again. So God, why did you make me dumb enough to start smoking after I lost the addiction? Sorry, I'm not blaming it on you.

Yep, after four years of smoking, I gave it up for another six years and by that time I never even thought about a cigarette. People could smoke in front of me and even blow smoke in my face and all it did was tell me how bad it smelled. I would have never believed smoking would ever come back into my life; but nooo! It came back in such a fierce and sudden way, I don't think I even realized it until it was far too late.

I think I have to blame my relapse on an unhappy home and in your face fights between a loveless couple; Na, come to think about it I have to blame it on me and nobody else. But it happened like this: As I partly explained, one day after a fight you don't want to waste time remembering, my wife stormed out of the house leaving her pack of Virginia Slims on the coffee table. For some stupid reason I felt, "What the Hell. Since she left them, I think I'll have one." God, what a mistake that was! It's times like those you wish you had a time machine so you could quickly undo your life altering screw-ups.

Without hesitation I pulled one of those long skinny smokes from the pack and lit her up. My first reaction was total shock on how good it tasted. I told myself several times, as I puffed heavily, I didn't remember cigarettes tasting so good. And I mean I was sucking on that thing so hard and fast I swear the cigarette glowed cheery red with the ash on the skinny smoke reaching two inches long and consuming almost half of it. I really had that baby fired up and glowing as I continued to think about how really good it tasted; but then it hit me. The room started to sway as I got dizzier by the second until I could hardly stand up. I'm not sure because I didn't have a mirror, but if a sick feeling ever made you feel green, then brother, that day I must have been a deep dark shinny green.

As I banged back and forth on the hall wall trying to reach the bathroom before upchucking on the new carpet, I kept asking myself why I can be so dumb at times, and man, I felt this was one of those times. I grabbed that toilet bowl and began driving the porcelain bus like I was on the highway to Hell in the Peruvian Andes. I betcha I threw up some of the donut I ate back when I was driving to my first class in college. I'll tell ya this for a fact, if I've ever been sicker, I can't remember when.

Now, after getting rid of that last little piece of graham cracker from kindergarten, I stumbled to the living room and flopped on the couch like a bundled up and sopping wet, two hundred pounds of rags.   The swirling bed spins had me believing I just consumed a fifth of Old #7, and bed spins were, and are, one of my most reviled feelings. From the first moment to the last moment of this ordeal I kept cussing myself for being so stupid. But thankfully it wasn't long before I drifted off for a good solid two hour nap. When I woke I was thankful the nausea had left me, but I was still angry about what just happened. I'm sorry to say the funny part of this whole thing, or maybe I should say the most terrible part of the whole thing, it was less than a half hour after I woke from my nap, the terrible urge to have another cigarette was overpowering. When I say overpowering, I mean I wanted I cigarette like I never quit smoking; that's how overpowering it was. Five years of never even thinking about a smoke and now I want one as if I was smoking up to yesterday.   I would have never believed it if I hadn't felt it myself first hand. The idea of going five years without and now wanting one was beyond me.

So, of course, I had to have another cigarette, but this time I wouldn't suck on it so hard. And yes, it tasted just as good as the first time. I felt bad about what I was doing, but I don't know if it was just my poor state of mind at the time, or if I just didn't give a damn and I wanted a cigarette. Is there a law against that? I doubt it; but if you ever quit smoking and started again, by golly, there should be a law. If there was, I wouldn't have smoked another decade before finding the balls to give it up again. And for me to quit it took humongous balls. The first three weeks were like somebody constantly squeezing your insides and every time you see or smell a cig the squeezing becomes so tight and the chills so cold you wonder if you can keep breathing at all. From three to six weeks it was a constant nagging; a constant wanting of something you banned and every minute of the six weeks you wondered why you banned it. From the six week mark I wanted a cigarette for the next six months, but the urge wasn't knee weakening or cold chill shaking like the first six weeks. The urges were controllable and you sure didn't want to blow it after six weeks of pure hell. After six months occasionally you would get an urge, but it was more of a nuisance and a pain in the butt, than a pain in the gut, from the sweet addiction of nicotine.

I pulled from the memory of how hard it was to stop smoking when I focused on the little jars of medicine sitting there in front of me. I started wondering about the cause and effect of this stuff and if it was going to make me want a cigarette like the last time I put smoke to my lips. If that was the deal, then I say no thanks to any of this treachery. I've been off the smoking scene for decades now and I never want to go through the process of throwing the monkey off my back again, much less supporting a five dollar a pack habit. When I wanted to quit I told myself I'd do it at two dollars a pack. I didn't get it done until they were two-ten a pack. Five dollar a pack cigarette sounds as bad as one hundred dollars for seven grams of weed. Let's see, five dollars times thirty days equal's one hundred fifty big ones. Wow, one-fifty a month sounds terrible and I'm thinking about buying smoke that costs three hundred plus a month. It seems like I have two little men standing on each of my shoulders constantly whispering in my ear. I wonder why they tell me the exact opposite every time they yell at me. Well, I think I'm going to listen to the one who tells me to watch out for any wayward monkeys looking for a home; not on my back ever again. I'm not sure anything is worth shooing a monkey off your back.

Now that I just remembered the hard time with smoking, I then started thinking about hard times with drinking. I have to say I never really had a drinking problem because I was so against it; or so I thought. Oh, back late in my first marriage I started enjoying a little Johnny Walker Black Label Scotch every night after work. Scotch is one of the spirits I can say I truly love. I'll drink vodka and bourbon, but it doesn't do anything to me like a little Red or Black Label. Since I really couldn't afford those two labels, I have never even tried the Blue Label. That's for the Rockefellers of the world not the working class man like me.

When you enjoy drinking liquor on a regular basis, there is much more in it than just the sip. You have to have the right size glass to hold the crystal clear ice cubes you must purchase at the store. Refrigerator ice just won't cut it. How can you pour that beautiful amber liquid over milky and pitted ice? Not for Johnny Walker you don't. He demands the respect of pure crystal ice in the right goblet to give a melody of synchronized clinking as the ice swirls around the glass. Of course the sip and the warmth of the amber going down is the payday, but the whole symphony of all the parts is what a drinker thinks about; and that's what I thought about. Every day around four o'clock I started thinking about the soothing liquid flowing softly over crystal clear ice making a sound as welcoming as the whop, whop, whop of a helicopter to a Marine in the field. And I must say when I started dreaming for a glass of scotch at four in the afternoon while I'm supposed to be focused on work, I knew for sure it must be time to look in the mirror and see if a visitor crawled on my back and surprised me when I wasn't looking.

I spent several days thinking about what was happening with me and Mr. Walker. I thought about it and then I went home and drank it; and I did that about four days before I decided there really might be a monkey on my back. I didn't think he was a large one, but I didn't want him to grow up at my expense, either. He may have a small grip on me, but it didn't seem he had his nails dug in so far they would have to be surgically removed. I was about twenty-nine years old at the time and I didn't want to go through life wanting a glass of scotch at four in the afternoon; and I sure didn't want to go home and drink till bedtime. So, that night I went home and poured a more than half full bottle, of what I think is the best Scotch going, right down the drain with all the other rejects and unwanted's.

I have to admit pouring out such a pricy concoction was a very hard thing to do. At the time I believe I was paying about fifteen bucks a bottle when I was making about five bucks an hour. I made economics a major argument for giving it the drain. I believe the same bottle is around forty bucks today. You have to pull out three one hundred dollar bills to get into the Blue Label area of sipping and now we're getting back to the price of medications al la cannabis.

But, pour it in the drain I did and I spent the whole night cussing myself for doing it. Actually, I spent the next two weeks cussing myself. Why didn't you just finish the bottle? It's almost sacrilege to dump such finely distilled spirits down the same place toilet water goes. Good Scotch must be run through the human body before it ends up in such a demeaning place as the sewer. Well, when I started telling myself bullshit spin like that, I knew Mr. Primate may be a little bigger and have nails just a little longer than I imagined. And on that twenty-ninth year of my life I gave Johnny Walker a fond kiss good-bye. I will say, on very special occasions, I may flirt with a taste of Mr. Walker, but usually when I think about it, the special occasion doesn't seem all that special considering how much that son-of-a-bitch wants me. It takes a daughter's wedding or the defeat of some incompetent president for me to have the liquid pored; but those times come very rarely, thank heavens. I'm also thankful the scotch doesn't have the same effect as tobacco. Today I can go out and have a drink of bourbon or a nice martini with three olives and never think a thing about it; but, as I write this the only spirits I have in my home is a bottle of Jack given to me when I left work; it is unopened and it was given to me almost three years ago. Since I was thirty I prefer ice tea, coffee and an occasional beer when a couple of buddies come over to watch a NASCAR race.

Obviously I knew what an addiction was and how hard it is to stop doing something you love; and that covers everything from, tobacco, alcohol, food, sports, TV, hobbies and probably the hardest; women. (I shouldn't put women in this lousy category; I'm sure women feel the same about men at times.) My main concern, will I place medical marijuana in this not-so-majestic category of other monkey loving addictions? Because, if there was a chance, I knew about the demon and I never wanted another one on my back as long as I live. I will sit around in major discomfort before I let that crap happen to me again. No way, no how, no nothing will let me knowingly allow anything to control my life but air, food, water and that's about it. (Love if I can ever get it).

"Oh, boy," I said to myself in total mystification, "this thing has happened so fast I didn't take time to think the whole thing out." And, believe me, I really didn't. Sitting there staring at the two jars of pot and all the paraphernalia needed to use it, I think I felt more like a illegal stoner than a patient who needed a particular medication to give relief for a certain malady. And that got me thinking even deeper. My mind went to my parents and especially my Mother. Some call her my Step-Mother because my Father married her after my natural Mother passed; but I love her as much as any Son loves his Mom, therefore she will always be called my second Mother or my other Mother. But anyway, now that she is in her mid-eighties her medicine cabinet looks like the CVS pharmacy right after the daily delivery. There are so many medications for my poor Mom you literally have to have a Microsoft document printed out with check mark spaces to make sure she gets whatever she needs on the right time of day. And with all those medications in the cabinet, were any of them better or worse than the medication sitting in front of me? Did any of her, or my Father's, medications put a monkey on their backs? I don't know, maybe when you're eighty-five with your own maladies it may be possible monkeys don't mean as much as they did when you were twenty-five.

I had just spent quite a while pondering the torment of kicking the addiction of tobacco and the love of Scotch; but I also remember putting down a good quantity of weed in my college days, too. Now, you have to understand sometimes it's hard for me to remember what I had for dinner last night, so you may want to take this next statement for what it is; just a faded memory. And my memory remembers if you had it you smoked it and I mean you smoked it heavily until you ran out. If you couldn't find pot for a few weeks it might have been a nuisance for a couple of days, but, by the time you found, or could afford, you next baggie, I don't remember ever being extremely wanting for it like I was with tobacco or Scotch.

I do remember I was once scheduled for a job interview in a week or so when my brother-in-law from my first marriage stopped by with, what he called some killer weed. Since I had to give up smoking about two weeks before so I'd be sure to pass the drug test, I had to stand out on my porch and look in as he and my wife partook in taking turns kissing a bong. If I remember right, and I'm sure I do, I was more upset I was standing out on the porch to prevent contact contamination than from messing up any drug test even if the interview went that far; but I'm sure I didn't get the squeezes and cold chills like I did when I saw somebody puffing on a cigarette.

The thought was very troubling for me. Was I right in my remembering? Could I use this as a legitimate medication to help stop the tingle and promote restful sleep? Do I have to worry about a very hard addiction battle and is the battle ahead worth trading for restful slumber? Right or wrong I decided I would use the product in front of me and see what kind of reaction I would have when it was gone. If I really had a craving when the bottles were empty, then I better reevaluate the situation. Since it was mid-day Saturday and I was tired from all the running around, I decided to take a nap and check out the quality of the strain later that night.

Chapter Five: *First Use.*

I have to admit I was looking forward to bedtime to see if the weed the Budtender recommended would meet all his high expectations. After a fairly relaxing day I didn't think I needed medication on this particular night, but my curiosity was definitely getting the best of me and I was eager to give it a try. I decided I would keep my smoking to the bedroom to keep the aroma out of the front area where may friends gather. I remembered having an old valet box with a flat area, a little drawer to hold everything, and an area that held the little jars like it was made just for my personal medicating needs. You might say it was my very own doctor's bag.

The joint Nameless gave me was about five puffs per half so I thought I would give this weed about five puffs to compare with the previous. Since it was nine and bedtime was usually around ten, I ground a small part of a bud and scraped it into a pile on the flat area of the box. I took the ace of spades out of a box of cards and sat it beside the Bic lighter and the little glass pipe that were lying right beside the pile of meds. Since it was bed time and Indica was another way of saying indoors, whatever that means, it was the Sweet Tooth I had ground into the pile. I filled the corner of the card with finely ground weed and poured it into the bowl and brought the pipe to my lips. With a deep sigh on what I was about to do, with a strike of the lighter the flame engulfed the weed until the smoke disappeared into my lungs as the weed disappeared into the lower bowl in a fireworks show of sparks and pops. As I held the smoke deep in my lungs I loaded up the corner of the card again and continued the same process until I reached my goal of five puffs. Several puffs sparked off a chocking attack that I tried very hard to hold in and not cough out a very expensive multi-dollar a puff. But within the five puffs I found out quickly how much and how deep I could draw before I was reaching for the glass of water to quell the coughing attack.

I must say I was very surprised on what little amount I used for 5 puffs. It was probably more like an eighth of a doobie or even less compared to the doobie Nameless gave me. Since it seemed like such a small amount used, at that time, I wondered if I was going to get the same effect as my friends smoke gave me. I also took note of the sweet and fruity taste the puff provided me. I had never tasted such a sweet smoke and it started me wondering if the sweet taste was just a means of cover for a very bitter monkey. Either way, I remember thinking what a perfect name it was; Sweet Tooth.

I put the doctor's bag aside and settled in to see what would happen. I'm not sure "see" was the right metaphor. Let's just say the Nameless weed relaxed me and took away at least half the tingle and most of the burning in my arms. You ask how this weed reacted to my arms? I can only answer by asking, "What arms? I'm supposed to have arms? If I do, I sure wouldn't know where to find them on this particular minute!" Geez-o-flip I couldn't believe the stone that just walked up and hit me on the back of the head with a sledge hammer. When I was doing some research they talked about a term I didn't understand at the time I read it; but I certainly understand it now. The term was known as "couch lock" and even though I was sitting in the chair in front of my computer, it might as well have been a couch because I was a locked to the chair as if ropes we tied all around me. This was a high far more intense than I ever expected.

The only thing to ever affect me more than five puffs of Sweet Tooth would require taking a

trip back to my late twenties. This weed provided
the perfect medium to get there; but I was so stone
and un-expecting; you might even say scared, I was
wondering if I let myself go there would ever be
able to get back.

I couldn't stop my mind remembering when
a young man's back would give him endless
problems. Unfortunately, the young man was me.
It wouldn't take much to send my back into nagging
pain, and every so often, it would take me down for
the count as it did one particular October day. My
back went out so bad it was pure torture just to get
up and go to the bathroom. It was then I realized
how helpless a baby was because it seemed like I
was the baby. I mean, I couldn't even move my
little finger without feeling like someone shoved a
K-bar deep into my lower back. I was as helpless as
any new born baby. When it reached the point I
couldn't get out of bed to go to the bathroom, my
wife dragged me yelling and screaming to the car
and on to the emergency room. I guess the hospital
staff knew what kind of pain I was in when they
tried to pull me from the car. I imagine the people
within a half mile thought somebody was slowly
being murdered; which come to think about it, it felt
exactly like what was happening. Up till then I
would have never thought a pain could be so
intense. They say a woman's birth is about as much

pain as a human can stand. If that's true and birth gives more pain than my back ache, I'm wondering how any family has more than one child.

So, they got me into a wheelchair and wheeled me into the hospital and left me sitting there in front of the television. It just happened the World Series was on and Vin Scully was calling the game between the Dodgers and the hated Yanks. (Remember, I'm from Southern California) I think the year was 1978, but I'm not real sure so don't hold it to me. If you're a baseball fan you know and if you aren't it don't matter. Anyway, before I knew it a nurse was there with a shot of morphine being squirted into my arm. I'm telling you with no exaggeration, I felt the juice run up my arm, across my shoulders and into my neck before it swirled around my brain like a tornado on a mission; and it didn't seem like the mission was very darn secret. I couldn't believe how fast this stuff reacted and what a total euphoric feeling it gave me. By the time she removed the needle, I have to say my back hurt just as bad, but I didn't even give a damn; and I mean I didn't give a damn. I closed my eyes and listened to the game until I was literally sitting behind first base in Yankee Stadium watching the game as Vinnie gave the play by play.

I don't know how long I was sitting there when the doctor pulled me from the game, but my first words to him were, "Doc, I can see why this shit is illegal. If it wasn't, the world would be a stoned faced vegetable garden." He didn't seem too humored by the statement. He just told me it was a very serious medicine and it shouldn't be messed with until its absolutely necessary; and at that moment, it was absolutely necessary. But still, I'm very thankful I never got offered this crap when I was younger and dumber. With my addictive personality, if I had, I'm sure I wouldn't have stopped until I was as dead as King Tut.

Four hours later when the magic elixir was starting to wear off, I found myself wondering if I could go back and get some more. Of course I didn't, and thankfully, I must have grown out of my back problems because I don't have near the problems as I once did. But now I have another problem and I'm sitting here stoned on my ass trying to medicate against it. Hmm, I wonder if this is the way to go, but it seemed like I was wondering about everything and how everything affects every other thing. My God it seems like everything is so confusing and it was obvious, even to the stoned me, I wasn't used to being this high. Heck, I wasn't used to any kind of high or much less on how to control it; or, should I even try to control it? Maybe I should just relax and let it run its course and not try to evaluate all my thoughts. But on the other hand, this is what it's all about; the evaluation of medical marijuana and the cause and affect it has on me.

Boy, it was obvious it had an effect on me. My problem was I didn't know what the cause was going to be. As I sat there locked to my chair, my attention went to my dog Samantha. Like always, she was curled up on the bed with her head on my pillow. She never slept in the bed when I was in it; I mean you have to draw a line somewhere; but when I was at the computer it was a normal thing for her to curl up for a dog cat nap. I remembered how cute I thought she was curled up in blissful sleep; but just as fast, I wondered why a dog was on the bed. My Mom would never have allowed dogs in the house much less on the bed; should I? Then I got to thinking about it. Samantha has been curling up on my bed for the last nine years. In my house it's always been; if you don't like pet hair don't sit on the furniture. I never thought a thing about her being on my bed before; why should I think about it now? I guess I shouldn't be thinking of such things; but the funny part; I was. I was thinking about it and everything else in-between thoughts. It seemed my mind was gong a thousand miles an hour and trying to find an explanation to every shortcoming of life itself. Boy was I stoned. The Budtender told me Indica was a body stone and darned if he wasn't right; but, he also said Sativa was he head high. But come on, my mind is going mach one so what is the Sativa going to be like? I better not try and analyze Sativa until I can get a small grip on Indica.

Since I was so couched locked I thought I better see what it was like to stand up and walk. I'm not kidding when I tell you I didn't think I would be able to; but I gave it the old college try and up I stood to go into the living room. I was really surprised when I didn't bounce off the hall walls like I would've if I was this messed up on alcohol. The high seem more of a body thing than a mind thing. My sight wasn't blurry or double versioned like you would get under the influence of booze and my hand-eye coordination was a little off, but nothing like being drunk. It seemed like the Pot was affecting my mind and thinking process, but not affecting the communications from the mind to commands affecting the bodies functioning abilities. In other words I was surprised I didn't stagger down the hall to the living room.

I also had a small toothache at the time and I tried to evaluate the effect on the pain. I concluded there was not much analgesic power to it, but it was closer to the morphine's ability to make you not give a shit. It wasn't close to being as euphoric as the morphine, but I must admit, I was feeling pretty darn good and my tingling arms were the farthest thing from my mind. And because of that very large fact, step one of the process seemed like it was a roaring success, but I also knew this was just the very beginning of the steps to learn more about this thing known now as medical marijuana.

One thing I didn't know about Pot I was about to learn very quickly. This morning I thought I was going to buy some medical marijuana. I had no idea about Sativa, Indica and hybrids. I didn't know the strains gave different affects and even different varieties may change the high. It seems the breeders have intensified the high with countless varieties of Sativa and the same amount with Indica's and hybrids. They've given them names such as Urban Poison, LAPD, Purple Voodoo, Fruity Thai, White Panther, Candy Kush, OG Kush, 8 Miles High, Medijuana, Yumbolt and probably a thousand others; each with a supposedly different high and effect. The highs are said to come in the range of positive, social, relaxing, uplifting, melancholy, cerebral, creeping head, clear, active, paranoid and no panic. Now I want you to understand I don't profess to be any kind of expert on the subject, but at the time THC was THC and I had no idea Pot would give different affects with different types of weed, but it was a lesson I was about to learn real fast.

I imagine this would have been a
melancholy high by the way I reacted too it;
although, the fist use of such strong medication and
my inability to handle it probably had more to do
with putting me into such a melancholy frame of
mind. But it was certainly melancholy to me by my
reaction to the picture sitting on my living room
stereo cabinet. The picture is of a very beautiful
woman in her early forties and an OK looking man
seven years her elder. In the last ten years the
woman's beauty and facial characteristics haven't
changed a bit; but the man has become grey and
wrinkled with noticeable age since the time of her
death nearly a decade ago. When the picture was
taken the maladies and torments leading to the use
of medical marijuana would have never even been
considered; and just for that reason, I stood in front
of a picture representing the love of my life feeling
embarrassed by my condition and even worse by
feeling I had let her down. It was as if the eyes in
the picture were a direct line with heaven and in my
stoned and medicated first time, she was almost like
the cigarette I had all those years earlier; I needed
her as much as the morning she passed. As I gazed
upon the picture through tearful eyes it was if she
had died only yesterday. My grief seemed as strong
as it was ten years earlier when I stood in the same
place, starred at the same picture, and wondered
how I could live any kind of happy life without her.

Throughout my life I always looked forward planning on what would be. On that day ten years earlier was the first time I realized my yesterdays far outnumbered my tomorrows; and at the time I didn't even care about tomorrow much less ten years of them.

I knew I was in a previous time and I didn't like being there. Over the years I looked at the picture many times with fond memories; but it had been years since I felt the total grief I was feeling then. If this was the reaction I was going to get with medical marijuana, then I didn't want anything to do with it. No cure of any pain is worth bringing back life's greatest pain.

I turned away thinking TV might take my mind off my melancholy so, remote in hand, I sat down and surfed through the channels still thinking of her more than what was on the TV. It wasn't long before I was back to "couch lock" and totally engrossed in a comedy show laughing out loud with the audience. I knew I was over medicated when, about five minutes later, I realized I was on the Spanish channel and I don't speak a word of Spanish; but, man, did it seem funny at the time. Really, I hadn't laughed so hard since I don't know when.

I surfed through a few more channels until I realized there was much more going on in my mind than cold ever go on with TV. I just sat there for hours thinking about anything and everything; and I mean thinking about it in deep and profound ways. After what I thought was several hours of contemplating the world's ills, I figured I better pick it up and head off to bed. Again, I was very surprised when I glanced at the clock and realized only twenty minutes went by since I left my bedroom. To this day it seemed like the longest twenty minutes of my life.

Well, after contemplating on that for twenty minutes more; OK, maybe it was only twenty seconds before I thought I better get on to bed. But wait. My mind is going so fast; or maybe it's going so slow, that it seems like a million things to do before I turn in. I have to take my medicine, brush my teeth, let the dog out, get a glass of water, lock the door, turn off the porch light, check the front windows, turn down the air, turn off the TV, set the alarm, pull something out of the freezer for tomorrow night dinner…Wait! Wait one cotton-picking minute. How in the name of who knows am I going to remember all this? It's not like I do it every night, you know. Oh, wait another minute; I guess I do this every night without even thinking about it. Why does it seem like such a chore tonight

with a million more things to do? I started to learn
that very night the medication keeps your mind
spinning at one hundred miles an hour on one end
and spins as slow as a minute hand on the other. At
that moment I was wondering if I was going to
wake up in the bathtub and wondering why the tub
was in my bedroom.

Chapter Six: *Settling In*

That night, or should I say about four in the morning, I had to get up to make my usual pit stop. Again, I was very surprised to find myself sleepy, but I didn't feel anywhere near stoned. I went back to bed and, to my pleasure, slept till six-thirty. For what I bought it for, it worked. Sleep from ten P.M. to six-thirty A.M. is just what the Doctor ordered and I can't tell you how appreciative I was. But, on the other hand, I really didn't like the intense stone I encountered the night before. I liked my friend's milder meds far better. It seemed to work as good for sleep, but didn't put me in "couch lock" while doing it. However, there were a few points of the experiment that seemed promising. First and most of all I could look at the picture without going into the dregs, depression or the melancholy blues; it was just another day like any other and it was back to being another household fixture to gaze upon periodically. Second, there was no want for a regular cigarette, which pleased me very much; and third, I woke up fresh with a clear mind and ready for the day. That, my friends, is a very happy statement welcomed with both arms open.

There with my morning coffee I sat and pondered deeply on every aspect of the event as I saw it. But, geez, did I see it right? I loved the sleep part of the equation, but I sure didn't like the "couch lock". I remembered the Budtender telling me it might feel a little strong at first, but you get used to it up to a certain point. In other words he told me a person has to have a little time to learn how to handle this new and powerful stuff. I also thought about how my med was priced and sold as middle of the road cannabis; for crying out loud, what could the top shelve weed be like? It was very obvious to me I was a long way from needing that much medication. As I said before, being so screwed up you cannot get out of the couch comfortably is not my idea of pain management.

So, what to do? I thought at the time I needed a lot more knowledge than I had. I remember over-hearing the Budtender tell a patient a certain strain was about fifteen and a half percent of THC and since it was the weakest strain they had, it would be perfect for her daytime use. Not knowing much I figured it must be a Sativa. But if the Sativa I had was anything like the Sweet Tooth, I don't know how anyone could call it a med for day time use; or, you've built up a tolerance stronger than a male bull elephant. Since I don't have big ears and a long nose, I gave thought to going over and picking up some of the fifty dollar bottom shelf stuff just to give me a comparison. Since it was Sunday and they were open till noon, I decided to give it a try; but first, I have a little time to do some research on the web.

I did go get the medicine, but this time I went to a different Co-Op. I wanted a comparison so I thought I might as well go all the way with it. This place was very similar to the first place, although there was no six inch spiked red Mohawk as a Budtender. There was the same young staff of no more than twenty-five and it seemed they were every bit as knowledgeable. Along with the security guard and pile of paperwork only the strains were different; and even some of those were the same. I walked out with three grams each of two lower shelf strains and a super duper, high grade aircraft aluminum bud grinder with a lower gif catcher. I didn't even know what gif was, but it must be good considering the little two inch round thing cost thirty-five bucks. I was beginning to understand this medical marijuana thing was like all other healthcare prices; very expensive.

Another few days went by with only once needing to medicate. To my happiness the lower grade med worked more than just fine. It relaxed me and let me sleep without going through the "couch lock" phase. Since that day most of the time lower shelf meds were more than enough needed, but on occasion when the arms were really burning, I have to say, the stronger stuff works much better. I just had to make sure all was ready for bed before I partook. It was the medication and then the pillow. And to my delight I would never be awake when the 30 minute TV timer went off. Sometimes expensive things don't seem that expensive.

On the first day when I got home with my newly acquired medicine I was anxious to tell everyone I knew about my being a card carrying medical cannabis patient. After medicating a few times and having my mind think about every little detail at over a hundred miles an hour, for some reason, my mind had an abrupt and unquestionable changed. Did I want my Son and Girls knowing I was doing something I spent my life talking against? I don't think so. They grew up as hard working, loving, caring and responsible human beings and I'm proud of them. I don't want them to not be proud of me. Therefore, as of this writing, only two people know what I do and I think its better I keep it that way. Maybe next week my mind may go through another abrupt change, and if it does, I'll handle it then. But as of now it's my business and nobody else's. I guess if you're reading this I must have changed my mind.

Anyway, back to the walk into medical marijuana. A month or so went by until one day I went to a friend's for a long weekend. Of course I had to leave the meds at home so I was wondering what it would be like. Would I miss meds like I missed cigarettes? I didn't think I would but it took the three day weekend to prove it to myself. The only time I thought about medicating was in the middle of the night when I couldn't go back to sleep. Other than that I never thought once about the cannabis; that is until my head was on the pillow with my arms tingling and knowing I would not be able to drift off to deep, restful and dreamless sleep. I learned if I was to go away for more than three days I'd better take some edibles such as brownies or cookies or I'd be worn out and useless just like I was a few short months ago.

When I got home I was worn out and tired. My arms and hands were burning like I'd been out in the sun far too long. Not only that, bedtime and restful sleep was twelve hours away and between that time I was to have some company over. I didn't mind the company; I minded the dirty kitchen that needed to be cleaned before the guests arrived. Man, I wasn't up for it and I knew down to the core I wasn't up for it. I sat in my old familiar chair and thought about it long and hard. And then it came to me. I haven't tried the Sativa yet. They say it's the day time uplifting medication. I was used to the Indica's and if Sharks Breath is anything like that my guests will find me balled up in the corner sleeping as soundly as a Cheshire cat; the kitchen still in need of cleaning. But, since my stomach was a little queasy and I didn't think I would be able to down a pot of coffee for my energy boost, I instead went off to the doctor's bag to see firsthand what the Sativa strain was all about.

Since the meds had been sitting in the box for months, upon opening the jar, the fragrance floated from the confined buds in deep floral scents. Maybe there is a wine factor in this stuff after all. The smell was different; the look of the bud was different, and most of all, the taste and effect was very different. I knew right away this strain's effect was far different than the Indica I was used to. After sitting there for a few minutes analyzing the very fragrant and tasteful bud, its effect seems to be almost the opposite. I would have to tag this strain as a "dreamy" sort of feeling. If something on the news caught your attention you would soon be wondering what it would be like to be president of the US, Admiral Halsey or Paul McCartney. Unlike the Indica that lets your mind float all over the place, this strain seem to channel your attention down to one clear thought. The effect on the body was just as different. Unlike the numb "couch lock" feeling of the Indica, this strain kept your toe shaking quickly like a nervous habit, your fingers tapping the tabletop like you're bored and want to move on, and your mind trying to focus on something to fill it up.

I knew right away I'd have to be careful with this strain just by the way I attacked the kitchen. It was kinda like this: Let's see. I better wipe down this counter but look at the dirty microwave. That's disgusting. Better turn the radio a little louder. Yeah, the pictures are shaking, so that's good. I better move this appliance out of the way and clean under it and inside it; but wait; check out the dust on top of the Frigidaire. I wonder if the underneath is as bad as the microwave. Oh, geez, it worse. Since I've done this, I might as well clean the inside while I'm at it. Mop the floor, do the windows…This is what a good Sativa is like; or, I should say it's what it's like for me. Your intentions are to wipe down the counter and an hour and a half later your kitchen is sparkling like the hope diamond. Indica, on the other hand, is, "I hope there's a good old movie on TV or maybe a good ball game; on second thought, I think I'll just turn in."

And that's why I said I have to be careful of this strain. When I over do anything I pay for it later that night. While Indica says "go relax," Sativa says, "Let's polish the car". I sure didn't want these meds working against each other, so I learned quickly to be heavy on the Indica side and be carefully light on the Sativa side. I can't let myself forget I medicate for relaxation to stop the burn and tingle and to let me sleep much sounder.

That being said, I now have a clearer picture on what they meant by a daytime social and uplifting high. As I said earlier, nobody knows I medicate much less to say I'd been around people while under the influence. Although I was happy because I got the kitchen cleaned, I was still pretty medicated when my friends showed up. I must admit I was a little uncomfortable at first because I had a paranoid feeling they were staring at me because they knew I was high and upset with me because of it. I know now it was just a paranoid reaction from being unfamiliar with Sativa's effect on the mind. Twenty minutes later we were chatting and having our usual good time; however, it was commented on several occasions on how good a mood I was in. As of this writing several states are voting on legalization of cannabis, and if they do, I'm sure Sativa will be the choice of the recreational user.

As time moved on I became a lot more comfortable with the thought of using marijuana for medicinal purposes. In other words it didn't seem too much different than taking my cholesterol, ibuprofen, nortriptyline or the one a day vitamin tablet; it was just another jar of meds. But, I have thought more than once on the value of this drug compared to others. I believe the difference between most drugs, other than helping or curing a particular malady, most drugs do it without inebriation. This medicine is guaranteed to get you high with each use. The question is; is that good, or is that bad. I guess things like Yen and Yang, for every action there is an equal and opposite reaction, democrats and republicans, men and women, are just four ways to prove there will always be two sides to any and all equations. I imagine if you're not a user or never have been the answer to you will be, "of course not," or maybe even, "Hell no!" And maybe in most cases I might even agree with you. Let's call this equation one.

What would equation two look like and how can it even be considered? Well, maybe equation one has never had a continuing pain pounding on them like a hammer. Maybe they've never had nausea so bad it was hard to keep their head out of the toilet. Maybe they've never know the misery of getting only three hours of sporadic sleep at night after night after night. I guess if you've never had theses ugly maladies and many others just as bad, you wouldn't be able to understand or empathies. I try to explain it like this. A symptom that never lets you go for one minute, like the hic-ups for instance will badger you and badger you without pity. Imagine twenty-four hours a day of hic-ups. Obviously you could never be comfortable; not for one minute. You couldn't curl up in a chair and peacefully watch a movie or know you could find deep relaxing sleep when you turned in at night. All you could plan for is a continuing annoyance that will never give you a second of piece. Believe me, any annoyance that pounds on you week after week, month after month, will quickly turn from just an annoyance to a legitimate and sometimes unmanageable pain. Right now I certainly believe, if you're lucky enough to never have had a problem like this, you should fall on your knees and thank God every single day; but, I must also say, most people that do understand what I'm talking about thank God for the herb in their medicine jar. The relaxing properties of medical cannabis, no matter if it's the head high or the bodily stone, can serve the purpose of giving a sick individual just a little peace and relaxation.

You must remember, how something affects me may have a totally different effect on somebody else. What one strain does for me may work differently on you. Medical cannabis is listed to stop pain, reduce nausea, relieve glaucoma, induce sleep, reduce stress and help with probably twenty other maladies. For me, though, cannabis doesn't seem to be a pain analgesic. As time moves farther and farther away from my last epidural, the numbness in my hands increase as does the tingling; tingling as if I slept on my arms wrong until it gets so bad it's hard to lift my hand to comb my hair. The tingles and burning are there annoying me twenty-four hours a day; or at least every waking hour. After it gets to this point it's not too long before the true pain starts in my wrists and works up my forearms and all the way to my shoulders and neck.

When I get to this point, I know it's time for another shot in the spine. Why I'm saying this is because when the true pain starts, cannabis does not take my pain away; only the epidural takes it away. What the Indica does is help relax me so I don't think about the pain or brood over my misfortunes. I just seems to me it has a way to take your mind off the hurt; or, it has some way to disconnect the tingling in regards to sleep. I know it doesn't stop the tingling because when I wake up my arms are almost as bad as when I went to sleep. Without medical cannabis I can feel the tingle all night long as I stay in very shallow sleep. The Indica turns it off some way and allows me to fall in a much deeper slumber. Since I can only have an epidural four times a year or every three months, I used to be anxiously waiting for the three month relief; although I can't say I ever liked getting the shot. For days afterward my neck and shoulders ache and my head feels like a sixteen pound bowling ball being balanced on my eight pound weight limited neck. But since the last two weeks were usually so miserable waiting for the relief giving shot, which has a bad habit of making your whole life miserable, it was certainly worth giving up a few days of uncomfortable for a few months of relief. Now, I'm very happy to say, medical cannabis is allowing me to go four months and longer between shots; which is very fine by me.

Chapter Seven: *Learning More.*

As the months went by I became a lot more comfortable going in and out of the cannabis Co-Ops and a lot more familiar with the different effects from the different strains. I guess like most people that have a plethora of choices to choose from, I guess it's normal to have your personal favorites. What I soon found out about the Co-Ops was they didn't seem to have a consistent menu. Unlike a good restaurant where you know you will get a great steak or burger, form one month to the next your local Co-Op seemed like every item had changed. Being a member of four different dispensaries; although I only traded with three due to a large price difference, it seemed like the inconsistencies flowed across the board. Not only were they inconsistent, the effects between the strains were way off, too. From one store I could pick up a quarter ounce of "Blue Dream" with a strong effect and a mellow edge that did a great job for relaxing; then pick up what is called "Blue

Dream" from store two and expect the same effects. Instead, I'd get an uplifting rebel-rouser high that should be saved for Six Flags and all the thrill rides.

Now, I would never name names of the Co-Ops I belong to, but since none of them are there anymore, it probably wouldn't even matter; but I'll keep names to myself and speak about what I experienced. Understandably it seems most cities really don't want medical dispensaries in their cities so, one by one in my city, they're given a cease and desist order or threatened with court if they didn't close their doors. Most just went away from the brick and mortar stores; but they found a new way of delivery.

In the short two years I've been a patient, I have seen the Co-Ops change, the names of the strains changed, and there is still no clarity between State laws and Federal laws. Many cities have never allowed any cannabis store fronts within their borders; others have allowed them but have since changed their mind and thrown them all out. Yes, most cities don't want anything to do with them but other cities welcome them with open arms. The proof of the statement is some cities seem to have hundreds; literally hundreds. Again, I don't know what kind of system the cities have for tax collection, but the cities that allow them must be making a bundle. I have read the California law and the Attorney General's response on how to handle the implementation of the law and it seems to me it is up to the counties and cities to make their own laws on how they want it to be handled; they can accept it or reject it, but they do have to respect the rights the California law gave to its citizens.

Most of the walk-in Co-Ops are basically the same. Some are much fancier with a menu of forty items and more, while others are simple and basic with only a handful of strains. But with all my trips to the med shop I have started to wonder over time if this medical marijuana thing is more of a front for legalized recreational smoking or a real true to life place for medical needs. To tell you the truth I think it's probably somewhere around half and half. I say this because I've been in line waiting to get in the bud room when I heard a twenty year old kid call one of his friends on the cell and say, "Hey, dude, I'm at the club. Do you want me to score some for you? How much are you in for?"

To me this didn't sound like, or even look like, a medical marijuana patient. I see young kids bounce in the Co-Op and joke with the Budtender's like they were old smoking buddies. Every time I see a young kid with no apparent malady I always have to wonder what medical need cannabis is doing for them and what Doctor prescribed it. But, on the other hand, I've seen people with sunken eyes and grey skin barely able to walk in the place. I've seen them in wheelchairs, on crutches and leaning on people to get there for their much needed meds.

Over all I believe the Co-Op owners really believe in the medicinal value of cannabis; although, I also believe they are businessmen trying to make a living. If a kid comes in with a bona fide medical card approved by California, I don't think the Budtenders cares too much as long as the patient has spendable money. I will say I have seen an obviously very sick patient who only had enough to buy an eighth oz of bottom shelf weed, and then have the owner of the shop give him a quarter oz of the very best; a difference of almost fifty bucks. To say the least, the patient was very grateful. When the man left the owner shrugged his shoulders and nonchalantly said, "That cheap shit would have never helped that poor old guy." He turned and walked into the back saying to himself, "If I can't help someone like that, well, to Hell with the whole damn thing."

I'm not sure what the profit is on a cannabis Co-op or how much medicine they sell. I do know most businesses with a store front have to double their money to make it work. In other words, if a doll store buys a doll for ten bucks they usually try to get twenty bucks retail. In retail they call it a fifty percent markup (retail minus cost divided by retail) but in reality it's a hundred percent markup. I'm sure it's pretty close to the same for cannabis stores. If he sells a quarter oz for one hundred dollars he probably pays close to fifty; although I know the stores pay big taxes that aren't added to the hundred; so I guess that comes from his profit, too. Now, all this information has been picked up over time but nothing is chiseled in stone. Like everything else in this medical cannabis business, information is secret and guarded closely. It's a strange system I will spend more time talking about later.

Once, about a half year after I started medicating, a visit to the Co-op got me to really thinking. In one of the jars, Bubba Kush to be exact, I found a seed. Now, seeds in medical marijuana are a giant no-no. This is supposed to be sinsemilla not illegal junk smuggled over the border. I mean, after all, male plants and seeded females aren't even close in strength compared to sinse. When I asked the bud tender about it he told me occasionally a plant will stress itself and produce a seed or two in a hermaphrodite state. It's not uncommon and he told me, "Plant it! It may not sprout, but it's worth a shot."

On that statement I thought the guy was blowing some of his weed smoke up my butt; but no. He assured me a patient with a medical card is absolutely permitted to grow up to twelve plants. Now I really thought he was trying to get a giggle off a naive old man. Instead of making a big issue about the statement, it was more a realization I really didn't know a darn thing about the medical marijuana laws in the state where I live. And with that in mind, I went right home and looked up the California Prop 215 laws along with the State Senate Bill 420 section 11362.5 & 11362.7 and Assembly Bill 390. Well to my surprise, I don't know why I'm ever surprised when it comes to medical cannabis, the kid was definitely not blowing smoke out the bong; well, on this question at least. On the contrary, he was absolutely right on. The law has given the patient a right to grow twelve plants; which only six can be mature and harvestable. Six! I knew right away I'd have to look into this revelation.

I didn't have to think too long; I mean, come on. A quarter of an oz is the equivalent of seven non-filtered cigs that last for two or three week versus throwing a seed in the ground and get a pound of primo medicine? I want to look into this. I remembered I had a book on growing marijuana way back in the seventies. Being I never threw a book away, I climbed up into my garage rafters looking for the boxes of my old college textbooks. Boy, talk about a trip down memory lane, I'll bet it took two hours or more before I got to the book boxes. I saw childhood teddy bears, model airplanes, slot cars, school projects, old pictures and countless other things I totally forgot about. I knew at the time there were a number of thing being called by EBay and Craig's List; but eventually I came across the box marked books with big felt marker. Yep, under the political science and algebra texts was the little green book I remembered. The book is titled: *Marijuana Grower's Guide* by Mel Frank & Ed Rosenthal. Ed Rosenthal! This has to be the book; I mean...Ed Rosenthal is one of the giant names in the industry today. I've seen his names several times on the net and I even contemplated a purchase of his book at Barnes and Nobel. Yes this has to be the book.

As I read the book there were things that didn't make sense for even someone of my limited knowledge of cannabis. He talked about the male plants being not quite as powerful as the females; thus, the male plants should be moved to the far end of the grow box so the females could get the good light. That's adverse to everything said today. Male plants and seeded females are junk with less than one quarter the strength as middle grade sinsemilla. But then I remembered, back in the seventies there was no such thing as medical marijuana. Marijuana back then was grown for recreational users and stoners. Well, come to think about it, I guess not much has changed; has it? Anyway, thinking this book might be a little out of date I went on the computer and ordered his new book titled Ed Rosenthal's *Marijuana Growers Handbook* and continued with reading the old book. In it there was a little sketch on how to build a simple grow room that seemed to be just what I needed. Since grow rooms haven't changed since the seventies I went right down to Lowe's and picked up everything I thought I needed. I got the 2X2's, and the plywood, and the white paint, and the four foot florescent light fixtures and the accompanying four each of the four foot grow lights. I was right at one hundred and fifty dollars already but excited to get home and start a nice garden along with saving money; the investment was only a little more than a quarter oz of good Indica. Boy, was I inexperienced and about to learn some hard lessons.

When the project was complete it not only had the back corner of the garage all to itself, it had my pride and expectations on the crops to come. I did plant the seed I found, and to another surprise, it sprouted under the glow in the back corner; but it grew in a rapid and skinny way. So skinny, in fact, it couldn't even hold up its own weight. Since I was sure it was going to die, I placed it outside between to camouflaging plants in the direct sun. Again, the cannabis surprises came. That little plant stood straight up and its leaves became broad and green. I knew something wasn't right. Since it was a week since I went to the Post Office, I thought I might shoot on up and see if the new book had any information on what I was doing wrong and what the direct sun was doing right.

Again, surprise slapped me right in the face. Comparing Ed's old book to his new book was like comparing Chilton's Motor manual of a Ford model-A engine to a Boeing 787's jet engine. The book emphasized five major things: Lighting, air circulation/ventilation, nutrients, temperature and humidity. Geez, this thing is getting more complicated than I figured. My box doesn't have any of this except the lighting and according to this book my lighting is even wrong. The first book never mentioned metal halide bulbs with blue light for vegetation or the high pressure sodium with red light for flowering. I'm starting to feel real bad because it looks like I already wasted money; and man, I hate wasting money.

Alright, my little plant is doing well out in the sun and I can keep it hid from the gardeners for the next few weeks. Until then I better do a lot more research on how and how much theses five grow box necessities will be priced and managed. I have to say the surprises just kept coming. First, I looked into the lighting. According to the book and internet the definitive light for my 5X5X8 grow box size is a one thousand watt bulb; and that bulb has to burn for eighteen hour a day while in the vegetation stage and another twelve hours a day if in the flowering stage. At the time I didn't put all this together and that turned into another huge surprise; but more on that little screw-up later.

The 1000 watt light is so powerful and bright it makes a lot of heat. Because of that little fact you need a light housing with an exhaust fan connected to the housing to rid the box of excess heat. Don't forget about the small oscillating fan to keep the ladies wiggling and bending to help them grow strong at the trunk and branches while reducing the humidity from the soil and leaf evaporation. Just to make sure all is working together a thermometer and humidity meter is nice so you always know just what the level is. The last major items are timers to turn on and off the electrical along with an automatic thermostat to exit the heat when it gets too hot. Wow! That means I have to put two vents in my garage because it's hot enough already; one vent to bring in fresh air and another to remove the hot and used air. I say wow again. This is starting to look real expensive considering the bulb is fifty to one-hundred and fifty bucks, the housing is at least a hundred and don't forget the ballast. Oh, yeah, you need a two-hundred dollar ballast; one for each type bulb. Yikes! That's four-hundred big ones just for the ballasts. Yes, I need all of this plus an extra hundred and fifty dollars a month on my already high electric bill. I knew right then I was going to have to put this to the pencil to see if it made any sense at all to grow your own meds. I also knew either way it wasn't going to be cheap.

Chapter Eight: *Growing Green*

As I went deeper into the subject of growing meds I found many more things that would rid me of my money. I would need ducting for air circulation along with special made up organic soil for the ladies to grow strong in; not to mention planting pots of various sizes to match root growth. I guess if you're going to do it you need the super duper nutrients that come in veging and flowering formulations. Two parts for each formulation costing more than fifteen dollars a bottle; four quart bottles equal seventy bucks for all four. A Ph meter and a moisture gauge are two other necessities. Another wow! Will the cost of this little endeavor ever end? Another interesting surprise; even with all these costs I figured after a three or four month period to get my initial investment back, then, over all, it should reduce my med bill by half. I reasoned with myself I could also use it as a stress-less and interesting hobby. I mean after all, I have grown Orchids and African Violets for years now, so if I can handle that, there should be nothing to growing a weed. Now after being involved with growing for a while I can say it sure is interesting but I'm not so sure about stress less. Not knowing then there is a million things that can cause havoc with your garden; and in just a few short months it seemed I had to deal with most of them. Here's the story and how it evolved:

First I redid my grow box to today's technology. I installed the 1000 watt light along with all the fans, bells and whistles. I must say I was pretty proud when I stood back after putting the little plant under the massive light. I knew right away it seemed awfully lonely by itself so more seeds or clones were needed as soon as possible; so off I went on my personal cannabis hunt. Several of my Co-Ops handled six inch clones before but none of them had a single one. I finally found a store that sold feminized seeds. I was hoping to pick up several clones to give me a jump start on growing time, but I was happy to pick up the sativa rich Hashplant Haze and the Indica heavy Sour Diesel for the sleep medicine. I got six seeds of each at a price of fifteen bucks per seed. I preferred this to ordering seeds from Amsterdam via the U.S. Mail. It seems these seed banks ship all over the world, but at this time I just don't have the jewels to order overseas. Maybe I will later when I hear some more about it. One thing's for sure, the Amsterdam and Canadian growers by far have the most award winning strains. It's certainly something to think about.

The directions on the seed box stated the flowering time was ten to twelve weeks for the Hashplant Haze and seven to eight weeks for the Diesel; both with a probable yield of 500 to 600 grams. Let's have a triple wow! My brain went racing trying to figure it out. Five hundred and sixty grams is twenty ounces in any man's book and twenty ounces also equals a pound and a quarter in the same man's book. That's why I asked for a triple wow. If I could get twenty ounces out of each plant my med allowance wouldn't go in half, I would never be able to go through near that amount; in other words my cost would go down to the cost of electricity. Now, it was having absolutely no experience at all in marijuana growing that made me think the way I thought. And unfortunately, this is the way I thought: If I take a seed and plant it this week and next week I plant another seed and the following week another and so-on and so-forth, by twelve weeks the first would be flowered. I could harvest that one, take a clone from a younger one to save seeds and I would have a continuing garden with no more than the twelve allotted plants to boot. Boy that plan sure did sound good to me; and I have to admit I'm very embarrassed by the statement.

I must say it was very interesting and exciting watching the little ladies develop. For weeks all went as planned with all the seeds growing at different levels. It was also amazing how different each were to the others. Some were broad leafed and some narrow; some were deep green and some were lime green; some had seven fingers per leaf while other had nine. I couldn't help but wonder what the medical effects would be. I had vaporized enough to know a good strain from a bad one and I was hoping these would be the good ones; considering all the attention they were getting.

I was pretty happy with the results by about eight weeks in but the older plants didn't seem to be anywhere close to forming the big sticky buds as seen in Ed Rosenthal's book. Most of my reading was in the nutrient, vegetation and lighting chapters. Maybe it's time to read the chapter about flowering. Oh, man did I make a major mistake. I assumed the flowering time was the life cycle of the plant; NOT. I didn't realize there was the vegetation stage that had to come first, but my biggest mistake was thinking the plant would flower by itself. Wrong brilliant Bozo Grower; wrong again. The marijuana plant will not leave the vegetation state until the sun shows shorter days. After the June solstice different strains start to flower at different times; some in July for September harvest and others in September for November harvest. It was a hard lesson to learn, but now I know indoor growers go from an eighteen / six hour light cycle for veg down to a twelve / twelve hour light cycle to induce flowering. A little late but now the light bulb difference flashed in my brain. "Oh, that's what they mean by two different lights; metal halide for blue vegetation and high pressure sodium for red flowering. It's all coming crystal clear to me but what am I supposed to do now? I have ten plants in the grow room and they are coming awfully close to where the light will burn them. I now know what "sea of green" growing is all about. I have a sea of green with no buds and no more room to grow. The "book" says if you veg your plants until they are three feet tall you can expect them to grow at least another foot in the flowering state; a full third or more. Keep them in eighteen hours of light and they will just keep growing until the room gets too small or the light can't supply all its needs. Geez, why didn't I read the book a little more carefully?

Now what to do? I'm in a pickle with not too many options. I can't just change light and reduce time down to twelve hours. I would have ten plants flowering and maturing at the same time. I'm only allowed six mature plants and since I'm still uncomfortable with growing I sure don't want to break the law and lose my permit for medical marijuana. I did; I am; and I will always stick to the letter of the law of SB420. This is a very appreciative right and I never intend to knowingly abuse it. So what am I going to do? I can't just change lights and purchase another complete grow box pushing the thousand dollars mark; not to mention the usage of twenty eight thousand watts per day over whatever is now being used. Man, that's like leaving two central air conditioning units on most of the day. I know how everyone hates how high their electric bill goes in August; well, this is way worse. I was even nervous thinking about the power company checking on me to see what was up. I sure didn't want that hassle. This is supposed to be a stress-less hobby, remember?

No, I didn't want to run two units right now and there was no way I could put them out side. Every neighbor on each side has a wide open view with no place to hide; so, I had no choice but to destroy five of my plants and trim back the other six. With every snip of the trimmer I kicked myself twice for being so dumb; but snip away I did until the box was ready for the HPS. Yep, I had to dig out another three hundred and fifty bucks for a bulb and ballast. I must admit I was a little depressed with all the cash outlay and not even close to reaping my awards.

The change was as easy as screwing the new bulb into the same socket and housing and plugging it into the new HPS ballast. I was used to the bright clear light of the MH bulb so the orange'ish glow was quite a bit different. The plants must have loved it because in the next ten days I saw the first start of flowering and the little white hairs associated with it. All were beautiful females but the first one I planted; the male was the one I found in the Bubba Kush. Every grower has the same motto: No male's medaling in my garden of females. I'm the only male allowed.

Out of the grow box and into the spare bedroom went the lonely male. I kept it thinking I might try collecting some of the pollen for a possible breeding experiment down the road. I was thinking of a few other problems, too. I was now down to only five plants in the flowering stage with no clones and only a few seeds. It was a real hard lesson but I finally understood the simple rules on how to grow a medical marijuana garden when you're only allowed twelve plants and only six that can be what they call mature. To achieve this all you need is a combination of natural sun and artificial dark; or natural dark with artificial sun; or artificial sun and artificial dark. Understand? Neither did I until the time I was snipping away at two months work crying with pain on every snip;

trying to figure out what I did wrong and how I can remedy the wrong. Let me explain in simple terms what I came up with. In the spring time you can keep your plants outside without the worry of flowering or the cost of eighteen hours of 1000 watts burning up your meter. Come July, though, the days are getting shorter so some strains will start to start to flower. At that time you can keep six outdoors to complete flowering while you put the other six under eighteen hours of artificial light to keep them in the veg state. As you harvest one of your outdoor plants you can replace it with one from the grow box. Now that one will start to flower. You can keep this up until the sun changes position in the sky. Now you have to keep your veg plants outside so they don't flower and put the plants you want to flower in the grow box under only twelve hours of artificial light. The other way is to have two independent grow boxes with one burning eighteen hour a day and another burning twelve hour a day. In other words six of your plants have to be less than twelve hours for flowering while the other six wait in the vegetation room under the eighteen hours light. When you harvest the six that have flowered, you take six clones from the veggies; keep then under eighteen hours and move the adults into the flowering box. Now, you just have to be very careful to keep the clones alive. If these die you're back to seeds. It works much better to have your plants in different stages of growth.

I knew I had two very big problems. The first being I live in the city and not in the sticks or boonies. An ordinary track home with neighbors looking down into your yard is not what you would call stealth; not to mention gardeners, meter readers, cable men, linemen and telephone men crawling up and down the power poles. Even though outdoor growing is ten times better in regards to big yield, the security aspect is far from first-rate. So, growing outdoors is out for my particular situation. The other problem is the massive amounts of electricity used in a total of thirty hours per day for artificial lighting. I really didn't want to go into the substantial power drain that is needed for a quality garden. If you can't have quality there is no need for anything.

I really didn't know what to do at the time. It looked as if I would only be able to sprout seeds, give then two months vegetation and then another 8 weeks of flowering. This system only lets you grow six plants at a time and only a harvest of six plants every four to five months. Looks like the price of meds just went back up because this way of growing will not allow you to keep a continual garden going not to mention several other problems with this system of growing. The big one is finding

good seeds. There are very good seed banks in
Europe and Canada if you're willing to trust them
with your credit card number and getting the seeds
to you through the mail. Sometimes the Co-Ops
will carry them but it seems most are not feminized.
You definitely want feminized so you don't waste
plant space and light time on a something you're
going to trash. Regular seeds usually have a one to
one ratio of males to females; feminized seeds will
give you nineteen out of twenty. Even though
regular seeds sell anywhere from ten to fifteen
bucks and the feminized go from twenty to thirty
dollars, the time wasted with a male surely
outweighs the difference in price; my opinion.
Another problem with seeds is you may not know
what you're getting. Always go for the F-1 seed
over anything else. This assures you a close match
to the original strain. But even then, some plants
can be totally different from another. With seeds
you're just hoping you'll get a good one and it is a
very disappointing when it doesn't meet your
expectations.

Clones, on the other hand, will produce the
same plant over and over again. If you like a
particular plant, you can keep cloning it for years on
end if you're good; and I mean real good. The
cloning technique is very easy but you need to be
very vigilant to be successful. It's done by snipping

a small branch from the mother plant and then getting the little bugger to grow. I happen to use a little root growth hormone but some don't like this way. If I could cut three or four from each plant it would insure one or more would survive; however, when you can only have so many plants in your possession, the root hormone increases your chances for success by a wide margin. Even then there is no guarantee the little plant will live. I found most like to be misted several time a day so the leafs can absorb the water until it can develop its root system. I've had clones look good after two weeks and then kicked the bucket in a month's time. Usually, if you can keep them alive for three weeks you have the ballgame won. Your little plants destiny will be for large, beautiful, and sweet smelling buds just like its mother.

Since I had a couple of months before this crop should be harvested, I figured I had some time to think about my dilemma and how I should go about handling it. A month in and I still had no idea. It was about that time I called my nameless friend and eventually we got on the subject of growing. To my surprise, he had been thinking of growing but he had the same concerns as I; but, since he needed a lot more meds than I, he was very interested in reducing his med bill. And just like I was a few months earlier, he really had no clue on where to start or what to do. Since I spent most of the last two months studying as much as I could get my hands on, which is an unending amount across the web and U-Tube; I could help him through my own pitfalls.

Unlike me, he lived on a lonely street with a large flood canal wash on one side and a bigger hill, almost a cliff, on the other side of the lonely road. His property was long and narrow with a home one hundred yards away on the south side while the house on the North side must have been a quarter mile away, if not more. The entire backyard from property line to property line was a huge cement wash with fifteen foot concrete walls and a ten foot chain link fence at the very top. The access road for the flood workers was 35 feet away on the other side. Half the chain link fence was covered with a bamboo while the other half was bare due to the bamboo slowly disintegrating. I knew in an instant, with a little time and money, we could build a secure enclosure in the baron North corner. It was an absolutely a perfect place.

Now it was time to talk turkey; or cannabis, if you will. With his property we had the ideal natural sun or natural dark depending on the time of year. I had the artificial sun or artificial dark no matter what time of year it was. Together, if we identified our individual plants, we could go to twelve adult plants and twenty-four veggies. Depending on the time of year he could have twelve plants in different stages of flowering while I had twelve in different stages of veging. When the seasons change, so will we. Now I will flower and he will veg; although, I knew we would have to be careful with veging outdoors. If we leave the light loving plants out in the spring and summer sun they will grow ten feet tall and far too big for my grow box. I have to flower at four feet to give the space to grow another foot and a half. My grow box is 5X5X6 and about right for the one, 1000 watt'er. I assured him, his 12 hour natural light would probably yield far more than my 12 hour artificial light. After our little talk we were both sure the partnership would work if we just split all the costs and rewards right down the middle; this would include electricity, nutrients, soil mix, grow containers, fence coverings and any other expense we might have. With a handshake we both were anxious, enthusiastic and eager to get started. At the time all we wanted was a crop that would supply both our medicinal needs and be at least as good as the store bought middle shelf strains. Yes, we agreed, we would both be very happy with that.

Chapter Nine: *Partners.*

It wasn't long before we sat down and planed out a rough system. Since Nameless was a lot more comfortable with his medical marijuana rights, he didn't mind at all in ordering a mix of seeds from Amsterdam. We thought Bubble Gum, Northern Lights, Medijuana and White Widow would be perfect to start with; a mix of both Sativa and Indica. Several have won multiple awards so we didn't mind sharing the one hundred and fifty dollar price tag. In the order we were also going to get five free seeds of unknown strains; but supposedly guaranteed to please. We'll see.

While we waited for the seed delivery we rolled up our sleeves and got to work on the garden's security enclosure. The four corners were 4X4 inch posts that were ten feet high. The walls were covered with that white, non-see-through, corrugated plastic sheeting that is mainly used for the covering on patios. We put a roof on using a solar-tex greenhouse plastic. We decided on a cover not only for security from the air, but also to keep the freeze and Jack Frost off our ladies on those cold January nights Between the roof and the side was a one foot opening all around the entire perimeter for good air circulation. The dimension was 12X16 feet which gave twelve plants their own 4X4 foot space to grow in. We both agreed it turned out pretty darn nice and even blended in to look like any other garden shed.

Since it was well into fall and I had six plants a few weeks into their flowering cycle, we decided to back the van up to my garage and take these six over to his house. Since there was nothing more to do, I planted my last two remaining seeds and cleaned the grow box in anticipation for the new renters. It was about three weeks when the new seeds from Amsterdam arrived. The seeds for each strain were in a little one inch zip-lock bags labeled BG, NL, WW, MJ, and ASST; meaning Bubble Gum, Northern Lights, White Widow, Medijuana and the assortment of the five free unknowns. Since the seeds were stealth shipped in a solar power brochure we named the plants Solar Power one through five. And after they grew it was interesting how every plant was different from the others. At the time I couldn't help wondering how different the effects would be.

While I was waiting for the seeds to sprout I collected the pollen off the male plant I let mature in the spare bedroom. After tapping the yellow pollen on a saucer I put the plate in a plastic bag and went over to Nameless' house to visit the girls. Boy was I shocked on how big the buds grew since last time I was here. I guess when you see something every day you don't see the change as dramatically. Anyway, since I really didn't know what I was doing I wasn't even sure if I was too late or maybe too early with this unknown procedure. On I went wetting a cotton swab with a little water and dabbing it over the pollen covered plate. I would then pick a nice bud about half way down the plant and swab the cotton over the little white hairs protruding from the sugary covered calyxes. I then tied a little red ribbon on that particular branch so we could know which ones were hopefully pollinated. I hoped it would produce seeds but it seemed there could only be a few weeks left before harvest. Time would tell.

I was way off on my time to harvest. My guess of a few weeks turned in to six weeks; a total of ten weeks in flowering. Legally we could have eighteen plants in vegetation, but my box could only handle about fourteen by the time they reached forty-three inches. The sea of green would eventually block the light for good solid growth. This is the time we transferred the forty-three inch tall plants over to the natural darkness for their final life cycle. Some plants reached six feet by harvest. Before I took them over I snipped three small clones from each one hoping I would get one or two successes. Later on we could decide which plants are to our own personal liking, but right now the game is to keep the garden in perpetual motion.

Later that day when I got to Nameless' I found the six flowered plants in the shed were taking up most of their allotted four square feet and it seemed each branch had a big, beautiful, thick and fragrant bud ready to microscope. It had just finished several days of rain and the air was crystal clear and clean. I learned one thing for sure on that beautiful day; flowering marijuana plants have a fragrance as thick as driving through Fillmore, California when the orange groves are in bloom. It's a beautiful smell if you've never smelled it but let me tell you; if this were in a housing track like my own any neighbor three houses down in all directions would know exactly what I was doing. Now I can understand why they sell those two hundred dollar air filters at the garden supplier. When it's my turn to flower I may have to look into adding one to my grow box.

With work to be done we rolled up our sleeves and began to transfer the new plants out of the one gallon pots and into the five gallon size to encourage larger root growth. Some say the twenty or even the thirty gallon is much better but we just don't have the room or the means to move around that much weight. Since the old plants were very near harvest, we pulled them out of the back section and replaced them with the newbie's where they would be out of the way. We both just about fainted when we saw the back three plants. We weren't quite sure what happened at first, but with a little summation from two very inexperienced farmers, we surmised the branches leaned up against the plastic walls leaving the beautiful buds to catch all the condensation and rain through the one foot opening. The sight was totally heartbreaking for both of us. Most of the buds on the back plants were like a head of lettuce you left in the Frigidaire far too long. They were gooey and mushy with a grey mold almost like spider webs all over them. Let's see, what were some of the rules according to the "book"? Was it something about circulation and humidity? Those poor back plants didn't get any of the one and got way too much of the other. They sat in their wetness slowly rotting; and it all happened with just a few days of rain.

Well, you can't smoke moldy weed. They say it's not very dangerous; but it can kill you. So, into the compost bin went most of our three plants buried in the back. We both knew there would have to be some changes made to the enclosure. After contemplating our mistake we took each bud and looked for mold under the 100X microscope; and any bud with even a glimmer of mold was cut off the plant with the entire branch. We moved what was left over to a corner of the shed and quarantined them behind a plastic curtain. A small fan was left blowing down on them for the next few days to dry them out and stop any more mold growth. After a few days it seemed to work because we saw no more signs of mold under the microscope; all we saw were those beautiful Trichomes we've been waiting so patiently for.

Trichomes are the little glands that grow on the surface of the plant to protect it from sun, weather and insects; but for the medical patient, it's where the good stuff is. This holds the main actor, THC, and most of the bit actors of the other cannabinoids. When it gets close to harvest some strains literally look like their buds have been sugar coated by Tony Tiger's cereal company. If you look at a bud under a 60 power loop you will see little polyps that look a lot like mushrooms with long skinny stalks and large round heads. When the plant first starts to flower they are quite small and crystal clear. As the buds mature so do the Tric's. They grow and go from the crystal clear to a milky white and on to rich amber. According to the "book", and it seems to be pretty right so far, when the Tric's go to the milky stage this is the right time to harvest if you want the clear head and uplifting high; better for the Sativa strains. While the closer to amber, preferably about 25% amber and 75% milky is more for the body stone and sleep; better for the Indica strains. As the plant ages the THC deteriorates and the CBD increases, this is when the Tric's turn amber. Most say there has not been enough research on the subject, but most agree the CBD cannabinoid some way is the controller of the THC; in other words CBD is believed to work with the THC to control the length of the high and the type of high; be it paranoid, happy, nervous, anxious, relaxed or sleepy. But, if the CBD is left too long it reduces the effect to the point of smoking nothing more than tobacco leaves without the nicotine. This is when the Madam is in her last spurt of life. They say there is about a ten day window for the highest and most potent medicine whether it's on the milky side or the amber side. You don't enjoy fruit when it is under ripe or over ripe and the "book" says the same is true about cannabis.

Well, now we're down to three nice plants and two that are cut up so bad they both together might be a quarter of the smallest of the three. So, we have three and a quarter plants after we started with ten. I don't think Ed Rosenthal would be too proud of us; I knew we weren't. But, there was still a lot to be thankful for. Of the three good plants one was ready for what she was created for; time in the curing jar. Now, I've learned growing weed is not like growing a weed in my vegetable garden; it's really hard to do and I still have a whole lot to learn. What I've read in the "book" and about a hundred places on the internet, drying and curing can be every bit as hard as growing and maybe even a lot more important. There are endless methods on the internet on just how to complete the process. I don't remember a thing about curing in Ed's first book back in the seventies and the first time I heard about it was in Ed's second book; but I guess for very good herb you have to cure it like a fine wine. The theory and process behind what a lot call the art of medical cannabis sounds simple, but like everything else in this little money saving (I hope) hobby, it's far from simple and closer to an art.

There are two basic steps in this process; drying and curing. The way I dry is with a 2X2 foot box that is four feet tall. I ran strings back and forth on four levels so I could hang a ten to eleven inch branches over the strings. I kept them close together but not touching. Remember circulation. Mold is a crop killer right now and you have to be aware every step of the way from here on out. Light is bad for THC so I use old Wall Street Journal's to lay over the top for darkness and the papers ability to absorb moisture. Now here is the first road sign you have to read correctly; how long to keep them in the box? You want the bud to be a little on the dry side. The leaves seem crisp but the stem doesn't break; it only bends with a half hearted snap. Now I personally trim everything before it goes into the drying box. Some people hang it with the roots and all the leaves on until it dries. I find it harder to trim when it's dry and crispy; not to mention a few other nice reasons I trim while wet.

So, when it gets to this stage of dryness is when the curing stage begins. I snip off all the buds from the branch and let them fall into a colored airtight apothecary jar big enough for the buds to fill the thing without being pressed down. Airtight is the dominant and most important word in the last process of curing. Usually there's not too much problem with the drying box if you have circulation and low humidity, but in the curing jar you're walking a tightrope with humidity; it's in an air sealed jar for heck's sake! But that's what cures it. It's what makes poor smoke good and good smoke great; on the other hand, if not done right, it will make great smoke taste like crap right up to ruining the whole growing season by forming a moldy mess. I knew this at the time so I played on the cautious side rather than lose the whole thing to Mr. Mold. Remember, when curing you're playing the line between slow drying and mold. It's that simple. The slower the weed dries the more chlorophyll is dissipated. Chlorophyll is what give grass its grassy taste and weed its weedy taste. The more you can draw out the better. Slow drying also lets the Terpenes (flavor and smell) meld and blend together deep in the bud. And believe me, that's the smell you've been dreaming about for five months.

But you have to make it happen and here is how you do it; or at least how you should do it. When those crispy buds go into the jar you leave them as long as you dare to. For me back then it was one day to prevent mold. When I opened the jar the buds felt moist and pliable again. What the jar did was to let the leaves pull moisture from the inside out. They say this also intensifies the THC. I laid them under the dark newspaper for a couple of hours and then back into the jar they went for another day. Then it was two days and as it dries I go longer and longer without opening the jar. The plant is using the air up and that is part of the process. The longer you can leave the jar closed without growing mold the better your herb will be. I have to say this takes experience and balls. But usually in two or three weeks the long and agonizing process is complete. You're very happy when you crack open that jar and let the smell of the sweet and fruity herb fill your mind in its own style of rush. As soon as you smell the sweet you know ya dun good. If, on the other hand, you get a whiff of nauseating ammonia, then hang your head and cry; your balls were too big and your experience too little. Oh, well, there's always next season.

Anyway, back to the harvest. Out of the three and a quarter plants, two were deemed ready for the trimmer; and the trimmer was me and Nameless. Now, the big boys have electric hand held trimmers and things that look like a washing machines that turns leafy buds into finely trimmed nuggets; all we have are scissors. It wasn't long before we both understood why the big boy's invest in these time saving inventions. Sitting at a table concentrating on cutting the leaves and not harming the buds becomes very monotonous, very fast. It's not long before the back aches, the eyes water, the nose runs from fragrance, every joint hurts and the left hand fingers and scissor blades are covered with a black and very sticky substance. Just about the time I was going to ask for a much needed break, Nameless said, "What say we take a break and try some of this finger hash?" And of course, I had no idea what he was talking about. He started rubbing his fingers together and it was like rubbing dried contact cement off your skin; it rolls up into a little black-like rubber ball. He then took his pocket knife out and scraped the goo off his scissor blades and then mine as he continued, "I read how to do this on the net somewhere. This black shit is the pure kief."

I certainly knew kief was the pure resin Tric's, but I didn't know it was them sticking to my fingers. When we were done harvesting the mini crop we both had three small rubber balls larger than a grain of kosher salt but smaller than a pepper corn. Now it was my turn to ask, "Are we supposed to smoke this or do we use it in your vaporizer?"

He shook his head back and forth with uncertainty. "I don't think I want to put this oily goo in my vape. It might melt down and light the damn thing on fire. I paid five hundred bucks for that overpriced thing and I sure don't want to see it go up in smoke." He got a big Cheshire cat smile and proudly said, "I saw a way on U-Tube."

I followed him into the kitchen and watched him open the Frigidaire, look at a mostly empty bottle of soda, split it between two glasses and then promptly cut the plastic bottle in two with the chef's knife. He pulled two table knifes out of the drawer and set them on the stove burner to get the tips red hot. He gave me the top of the bottle and told me to breath in when the ball of hash touched the knife. He held one knife under the open end of the bottle and dropped a ball of hash on it. The thing smoked a little but not enough to breathe in. Then he smashed the little ball with the other knife and a forest fire of smoke billowed from between the blades. Geez-o-flip what a hit! I had never experienced anything like it. It was the cleanest, sweetest and most powerful hit I had ever had. I returned the favor to him and then he returned it to me and I returned it to him again and when he started to heat up the last one I had to tell him I was no good for another. He smiled and thank me because neither was he.

We went back into the living room and flopped on the sofa. "I'm going to have to wait awhile before I get back to trimming. Right now I wouldn't worry about cutting off a bud, I'd worry about cutting off a finger." And I knew just what he meant. Then he said, "I'm thinking with a good cure, on any good exhale, this ganja will be able to drop a Moose at fifty paces."

I laughed at his joke and replied, "If it doesn't he'll be asking for a clone."

The Co-Ops list the hashes under the "extreme" portion of the menu; and they mean every wood of it. Nameless and I had to sit around for over an hour, not saying much, but enjoying *Gary Moore Live* on the CD. We both thought the extreme was perfect with a very good blues guitar, but we both agreed this is not, and shouldn't be, your daily med unless you know the door is closing on you. This sure ain't for kids. This is one hundred percent stoner zone and should only be used in the "extreme" situation. Finally, after an hour and a half we were able to get back to our work; although, Gary Moore continued to rattle the picture frames.

It didn't take long to notice if we cut an ounce of buds, probably a pound of sun leafs, sugar leafs, trim, stems and branches went to the compost. We found out later if you had an oz of wet buds you may not get a ¼ oz after it cured. At first this concerned me because we didn't come close to the 500 grams we were hoping for; we only got 280 grams, or 10 ounces of wet bud that dried down to four ounces dry. Hey, at the time that sounded real good to me. Two ounces at a going price of $100 per quarter means a savings of $800 big ones. Not only that, this top of the middle shelf will last me for months with another one and a quarter plants to be processed in a week or two. After that it will be another three or more months before the next harvest.

The program seemed to be moving right along. I vegged a few more and took them over for flowering. This is where I found the real difficulty in keeping a legal perpetual garden moving along without a hitch. When you can have plants numbering 24 veg or a mix of 12 / 12 it's much easier to garden using 24 plants over the individuals 12. The Ideal way is to have six flowered and harvested with another six in the veg state. Let's say I have three strains I really like or two plants of each strain in vegetation. You take two clones from each mother before moving her into the flowering stage. Now, if all your clones live you're running in high cotton. If only one dies, your veg is down to only five plants. If three weeks later one of the same strain dies you're down to three plants and one of your favorite strain is gone forever. Now you have to start back at seed and that can also be a tricky proposition if handled wrong.

Why I say that is because the new plants I took over turned into males. Unfortunately my friend didn't realize you could buy feminized seeds when he ordered and sure enough an even half of them turned out to be worthless gigolos. When that happens it reduces you plant yield by one sixth not to mention 18 or twelve hours light bill and possibly both for some growers. In other words, it's very expensive for several ways to let the male gender rape and pillage your garden. A feminized seed may cost ten dollars more but how much will a male cost your garden?

There are other problems to seeds just as there are problems with clones. Some growers will never buy clones due to the risk of bringing in another gardens pests and molds. Seed don't carry contamination. Another problem with the clone is it does not have a tap root like a seed; the clone's roots grow from the sides of the stem. A seed has a tap root that will head down and not stop until something like a pot stops it or it reaches it maximum. Therefore, it is said you should always plant feminized seeds when growing straight into the earth. Since potted plants have a restricted root system anyway, clones seem to do just as good as seeds when it comes to the five gallon containers. But the beauty of clones is you know exactly what you're getting; there's no hoping or guessing. The medicine will be the exact same every time.

You can't say that about seeds. Way back when a man named Mendel studies the common pea and today we know it as heredity and genetics. Since encyclopedias and full degrees are filled with this subject I won't even try to cover it here, but there is a small bit you should know about it when planting seeds. Mendel found when a plant with all type "A" characteristics mates with all B characteristics, the plant will produce all "A" in the first generation seeds, also called F1. The second, or F2 generation will produce three to one "A"; the F3 generation will be about six out of ten with the recessive gene. That's why growers want F1 seeds that are feminized. They know they will get the characteristics of the mother strain. When you play with the recessive genes you may get junk; you may get lucky and get something very special; but chances are… With only 12 plants there just isn't enough to risk on a lousy strain.

Growers usually try to breed three main categories into their ganja. First, of course, is the potency; next, longevity of the high; third, smoothness of the smoke. Those categories are on the medical and sellable side. On the growing side they want something that can grow fast; flower fast, and finally, to have tolerances against insects, molds and bacteria. For this reason I don't believe a small time grower has enough plants to experiment with the breeding of different characteristic. This being my case in point; remember I said I pollinated three buds on two different plants? Well, by golly, we got a total of 36 seeds from one plant and 12 from another. Haven't planted any of the twelve yet; but, out of the other, 3 of 5 seeds turned male on us. One of the two was lower shelf at best and the other didn't even make the bottom shelf; that, my friends, is called wasting time and electricity. My advice to you is let the large growers breed for the cannabis cup so all you have to do is pick up the seeds at the local Medical Marijuana Convention. If you make sure they're F1, I think most people find it much easier, much better, way faster, way cheaper; enough said.

So, that's the way we did it. We flowered outside in the enclosure from about mid October through mid March. We used April all the way to fall for veging. It worked and worked well, but in some ways my system held back productivity. At first it was no big deal because the supply was plenty for me. My only complaint at the time was we had more mid-shelf strains than top-shelf strains. I wanted to work on quality because the quantity was fine by both of us. But, as I said about productivity, the two systems were way out of balance. My system could hold only nine flowering plants shoved tightly together while his system could hold 12 plants with a 4X4 growing space. That's 12 flowering in large pots and more space than we need for veging in small pots.

It wasn't only space, but the outside plants would grow far faster and far bigger than my grow room ever thought of doing. My inside just couldn't keep up with how large and fast the outside would grow without a whole lot of experience and planning. It makes it tough to plan when all the strains are all different and grow at different speeds, heights and widths. This is where experience on what strains the patient prefers and why it's so important not to let the strain die when you find one to your liking. When you bring in a new plant it's the learning curve all over again. I have planted some strains four weeks before the next and in some cases the next flew past the first. When you have a strain high in THC and grows like that, then obviously that's one you want to perpetuate. To give you an example, from outside to inside, my five and a half foot plants may have 24 branches with four to five buds per branch with the top branch one large flower with many different buds clustered tightly together. When cut I may get four to five ounces that dries down to a mere one or two ounce. His plants in larger pots will grow two foot taller and more if I could veg them longer since they start to flower the minute we put them out. He'll double and triple my inside productivity. To say the least we both like the outdoor flower time much better.

Once when I wasn't keeping up and there was plenty of room, we took a feminized seed of Big Bud and planted it in the middle back of the enclosure in a nicely prepared and fertilized hole. We planted near the first of May and let that sucker live right there for its whole lifecycle. Wow, what a difference the outdoors makes. The enclosure was eleven feet tall and Mrs. Big took up every inch. It would have grown much taller but we had to keep trimming it back so it would have plenty of room when it flowered. But trimming it back made it much bushier and it eventually took up half the enclosure all by itself. It was two inches from the top and two feet from each wall. It must have had forty branches with a half pound of sticky and very fragrant buds on each one. For a cannabis grower it was a very beautiful sight. For two first time rookies it was almost unbelievable. That plant alone could probably last me a year.

So, as said, unless you grow only one crop a year, you need some kind of light system. But let me tell you, with plants growing to eleven feet high and almost as bushy wide, I couldn't see anyone going through that much weed even in a whole year's time; however, very few people could grow six plants that big unless you were far, far away from your closest neighbor. Until you smell it, you just can't imagine what a strong but lovely smell the good strains give off; beautiful to anyone's nose.

Needless to say, that humongous plant changed both our perceptions on growing medical marijuana. Mine went from hoping I could grow enough to supply my medical needs to wondering what I was going to do with all of it. I knew right then there was assumed pitfalls to an unlimited supply of upper shelf buds filling your med box. It's fairly easy to go through a measly quarter of an ounce of buds per week; if smoking, it's about seven cigarettes or one joint per day. That's one-hundred bucks a week; or four-hundred bucks a month; or four thousand eight- hundred great big ones every year. Unless you have deep pockets and the amount doesn't hurt your discretionary spending, most people become a lot harder on scheduling their medications when doling out that much money. When the box is full of an unlimited supply there's no need to limit or forgo one more fill of the vaporizer. Sadly I know people that can burn up an ounce a week and more.

Nameless, on the other hand, saw the gigantic bush as an entrepreneurial possibility; a way to get back some of our investment, if you will. Since I didn't want anything to do with professional growing this changed the direction of our grow operation. He wanted me to triple the size of my indoor by the margin of two, and possibly three, one -thousand watt bulbs. This didn't seem like a very good idea to me, but he had already talked with some of his old Co-Ops about supplying them with some of our surplus.

We met with two owners over at my house on a warm afternoon in December. We sat around, talked and watched football while getting to know each other. Since this business is so secretive and non-trusting a good relationship is essential to a successful affiliation. It was obvious the gentlemen were more comfortable with the situation than I was, but as time went on we all relaxed and became comfortable with each other. They gave us the complete third degree on our growing method. Since they wanted pure organically grown buds they did intensive questioning on fertilizers, plant media, insect suppression, veging and flowering time and on and on it went until it seemed we answered all the questions to their satisfaction.

It was then we pulled out our latest cure and let them both enjoy the fragrance as the thick perfume floated from the once sealed jar. We could tell by the smiles on their faces the first introduction was quite well received. Then they looked at several buds under the microscope and I knew by the shake of their heads was one of approval. "Looks great," the one guy said, "Now all that's left is to give it the med test. Do you mind if we light up in your home?"

Since I didn't, I handed him the bud grinder, forceps, a pack of cut corner Zig Zag, a rolling machine and a Bic lighter. I watched him closely as he ground the bud and started to roll one by hand without the aid of the machine. When he was done it looked almost identical to a store bought Lucky Strike. It was obvious to anyone who's tried to roll a joint by hand just how experienced this roller was.

He chuckled as both Nameless and I must have looked dumbfounded as we inspected his work.

We passed the joint around in what seemed to be way closer to recreational use than one of medicinal purposes. To say the least, the conversation got lighter and the football game got better. The conversation turned interesting when one of the guys asked, "You are recycling your trash, are you not?"

"If you mean marijuana trimmings, then yeah," Nameless answered. "We make sure every bit goes into the compost pile and not in the trash. This is mostly for security reasons seeing how much we have to throw away."

Both guys looked unbelieving towards the statement. They then tried to explain we were throwing away a valuable part of the plant. Even though the buds are by far the most potent, the entire plant is covered with capitates Trichomes containing the very valuable THC. He then described a system to withdraw the capitates called bubble hash or water extracted hash. He not only described the method, he showed us.

Since I kept about fifty grams of cuttings from one of my first harvests just because it seemed stupid to throw it away, the guy went out to his car and brought in what looked like four different colored bags. What I didn't notice was the fine mesh fabric at the bottom of all four; with each a different size. He put the first bag into a five gallon bucket, and then another and another until all four were nestled into the bucket. He told us the first in was a mere 25 microns; the next was 75 microns; then a 120 micron followed by the last bag of 220 micron mesh. He told us you can go up to about eight different sizes but he thought these four does the job.

Neither one of us had a clue to what the job was, much less what the bags were used for. He asked for cold water, ice and a kitchen hand mixer. Since I had all three he went to work showing us just what we had been throwing away. First he filled the bucket with cold water about half way up. He then put in some ice and a little trash on top; a little more ice and a little more weed until all fifty grams were in the bucket of ice and water. He then cranked up the mixer to high and began mixing the ice and weed like he was mixing pancake batter. He explained the ice would freeze the capitates and break them loose from the plant. After fifteen minutes of mixing, the mush looked like green bubbly goo; so called bubble hash. After it was mixed to his specifications, he swished the first bag up and down trying to force all the broken Trichomes through the first mesh of 220 microns.

The next bag, the 120 microns, was swirled around like the first. Since all the leaf material stayed in the first bag, the next bag had a film of a greenish colored substance that looked a lot like mud. He scooped that out with a tea spoon and spread it on the 20 micron drying sheet. The next bag was the 75 micron filter. This bag had far more substance in it and it was also lighter beige in color. Again it was scooped out and put on the drying sheet. The last bag, the 25 micron, had the least in it but he told us this is by far the most potent. It was very light in color and only filled a half of a teaspoon. Every bag from 120 on down to the 25 micron caught the pure broken off Trichs in the different size mesh. We got a total of just a tad over 10 grams out of the fifty grams of trash. At a retail of thirty to forty bucks a gram, it was obvious to both of us we had been trashing a valuable resource.

Needless to say we bought the bags right on the spot; one hundred and fifty dollars but we just saved 300 dollars in what we thought was trash and compost. Then the guy pulled out some of his own dried bubble hash for a try. I think the football game may get even better.

Hash is a pure hit of THC. It has a very clean taste but has a way of expanding in your lungs to set off an acute coughing attack. When you find out how much you can breathe without coughing, the rush to the mind and body is strong and immediate; after all, it's a pretty pure substance.

So strong, as a matter of fact, both Nameless and I were almost bolted to the sofa. We were both surprised when one of the guys wanted to walk down to the corner store for some munchies and drinks. When Nameless asked him how he could even walk to the door, much less to the store, he laughed out loud and told us both, "I've been using this shit since before it was a legal medical thing. Over the years I've learned how to Pimp the medicine and not let the medicine Pimp me. There's not much I can't do under the influence; and most things I can do way better."

At the time I didn't know if I wanted to pimp the medicine or even if I could by trying my very best. I knew one thing, I didn't really believe he was unaffected by such a strong drug and I couldn't believe everyone else wanted to go to the store in my condition; but off we went. The two blocks seemed like two miles. As a matter of fact, when we got to the busy store, I was a little paranoid thinking everyone there knew just what we had been doing. I was not at all used to being out in public when in a medicated way. As I studied the guy, he really didn't seem too effected by the hash. I was really having a hard time believing a person could smoke as much hash as we smoked and not be four sheets to the wind. It didn't take me long to believe just how in control he was.

I watched the counter man hand him his change when a quarter bounced off the counter and on its way to the floor. The guy simply kicked the quarter with the side of his foot like it was a hacky sack; it flew up to eye level as he held his open palm at waste level and waited for the quarter to fall right in his palm without moving his hand an inch. The quarter fell right in his palm as he closed his fingers around it. He simply said, "Thank you," as everyone around loudly applauded his dexterity. I don't think anyone there would have believed he did it after smoking so much hash; I sure didn't. Obviously, no amount of THC can Pimp this guy.

Chapter Ten: *Back on My Own.*

    Needless to say the meeting changed both our outlooks on growing. Nameless wanted to get much more involved with growing and providing the Co-Ops and I wanted just the opposite. I think we managed two more crops together before the final end came. Nameless not only wanted to harvest more, he wanted a friendlier environment in which to do it. Since he had a vacation home in Colorado, he set his sights for the mountains and the friendlier environment towards medical marijuana. I have to hand it to him, he knew what he wanted and he went for it; he went a long, long way for it. He rented his SoCal house and became a Colorado grower. The last time I heard from him everything was going toward his plans except one small detail. Colorado at the time of this writing is going to vote on the total legalization of marijuana and, if the vote passes, it will promptly put him out of business since the bill doesn't allow any sales. If it is made legal, will there be a need for medical marijuana Co-Ops anyway? Not only that, how will the Feds react to the will of the people? According to the Feds, Ganja is still a class one drug. Cocaine and other hard drugs only rate a class two in the Feds eyes. If the bill doesn't pass it's a moot subject but if it does pass then only time will tell what happens. If California votes down legalization I'm not sure anyone will pass it, but if they do, only time will be able to work out all the problems.

But, I was more concerned with my own problems. There was no way I would be able to grow outside and I wasn't too thrilled about two large grow boxes burning two thousand watts plus fans. The California law states you can have eight ounces of usable buds. When I first became aware of growing I thought eight ounces seem like a little much, but now I know for some growers it isn't. If you used one ounce a month you would need six or more ounces to hold you over seeing it takes that long to harvest a new crop. After growing awhile you will understand how easy it is too loose your entire harvest. Between powdery mildew, spider mites, soil gnats, white flies, black flies, forgetting to water, unbalanced Ph, mold, stressing the plant, too hot, too cold, too much humidity, too little humidity, and another dozen or so stumbling blocks, you can see how difficult it is to keep a perpetual garden, perpetual.

So, with six months' supply of meds on hand and a dozen veging clones under the 1000 watt metal halide, I had a big decision to make. I was back to hoping I could grow enough to keep me from having to spend four hundred dollars per ounce. It was even harder to take after growing some mighty fine ganja for one hundredth the price; although, I knew I would never be able to produce the yields of outside growing. Accepting that fact, I decided to go with two small grow boxes. The smaller would be a 3X3X6 foot burning a 400 watt metal halide for veging and a 5X5X8 foot burning a 600 watt high pressure sodium with two T-5 fluorescents kept low on the sides for thicker bottom growth. This is not much more than the one 1000 watt I originally used. With this system I can veg the plants to about 44 inches and transfer them over for bloom.

This system seems to work pretty well for me; although, the flowering process usually takes longer than the veging; especially with the Sativa's. This is why planning and knowing your favorite strains is so important. With such limited space you can't have plants waiting for the next phase. Even with a four hundred watt bulb the plants can burn if allowed to get to close. A thick canopy will also block light to the lower levels resulting in skinny, unhealthy, and low yielding plants. Excessive plucking and trimming can stress a lady into a hermaphrodite. Like all women I've ever known, they all do better when stress free and happy; and when their happy, I'm happy.

My yields have been very acceptable to me. I'm trying to keep the veg time for my plant about the same as the blooming; witch is around three months each. Optimal is plants in different stages of growth so you can harvest every few weeks or so; but, this is something that takes a few minutes to understand but years to master. I don't mind saying, I'm a long way from being called master grower.

I was so wrong when I thought medical marijuana was as easy as growing a weed; wrong! It is one of the most demanding undertakings I have ever been associated with. I believe one reason for this is the six month expectations you have in regards to potency and usability. If one of the tomato bushes doesn't do well in the garden it doesn't seem to be too big of deal; but if one of your ladies is struggling you're right to the internet to find out what makes the leaf tips go yellow and turn down. You constantly have to be on guard for all types of maladies. If any one of them is left untreated, the loss of the entire crop is a very good possibility. I liken a crop growing inside under the lights to my Grandfather's dairy farm. Those cows needed attention every morning at 5 AM and again at 5 PM. There were no sick days, or Christmas, or birthdays or even vacations. Those cows needed attention every single day; now you know what inside growing is all about. Plants need attention every single day. Most of the time, I must say, it's fun like any other hobby. But most hobbies can be set aside of a day, or a week, or even a month without any major problems. Not so with growing. If you're sick or tired the plants could care less. All they know is if you don't attend them you will lose however many months you have invested in them. It seems a little unfair that two months of hard work can be jeopardized with a few days of neglect. But, believe it. A beautiful garden can go south as fast as your tears can fall to the ground.

That's a major problem with growing. The optimal is to be linked with a very good friend to help with the farming when you need a vacation or want to fly to Vegas for a few days. But, now we're in a deeper quandary. I don't think the law will allow a non-card carrying person to tend a garden of marijuana. I'm not sure about that part of the law, but I know a card carrying patient would work better and be safer. You wouldn't want a friend busted for tending your crop.

And now we get into the security problem. I think everybody knows if you tell the wrong person the whole town may know about it in days or even hours. To a grower that's the last thing they want and/or need. The more secret your garden grows the better. Even if you're legal to grow twelve marijuana plants, if you're growing outside and the wrong helicopter spots you, you can bet you'll be getting a knock on the door; which in turn, will tell every neighbor what you've been up too. If someone outside the yard sees your crop and wants it, then you may have a much bigger problem than you think.

Back in the day, you know, when I picked up Ed's first book, a friend of mine built a greenhouse to grow a small crop. One day the cable guys were on the pole looking down in his garden. Since it was pretty obvious to what he was growing, my old friend had a casual conversation about growing thinking all was good. Not so. Since my friend worked the night shift it was his wife that got a knock on the door around midnight. Sure enough, there was the police with a report from the neighbors that two men were running through her yard and seemed to be dragging a bush. To say the least his wife was in shock and not knowing to tell them there was no problem there and to go away, she let them look around. The thieves pulled every plant up by the roots, but left enough leaves around to make clear her husband wasn't growing tomatoes. The only good thing about the ordeal was the police didn't take the guys wife to jail. This is why security is so very important. No plant is worth some idiot breaking into your house and killing your dog just so he can get his criminal fingers on your garden. Killing the dog is the best case scenario; we all know it could be much, much worse. Needless to say, security to a grower is a very big deal and anyone who knows about the garden should be a very good and trusted friend.

I guess if you're still reading you may be wondering if a walk into medical marijuana is right for you. If you are wondering then I feel bad for you because you must be near your ropes end; and I feel bad for anyone that's just hanging on to the ropes end. I wouldn't even attempt trying to talk you into it or out of it; I'm just saying how it is with me. If you are a person with limited means and unable to comfortably spend three hundred dollars a month, and maybe even more, then you should probably stay away from it. However, for anyone who decides to take the walk I strongly suggest you try to grow your own meds. At first, unless your thumb is truly green, you probably won't be able to produce top shelf ganja until time and experience shows you how.

Why I suggest growing your own herb is very simple, and in my opinion, very logical. After you're grown awhile you know the pitfalls on either side of the garden. Now, I don't want to imply to anyone I think I'm a master grower because I'm not. Like anything and everything there is always something new to learn and experience. That said, I do know enough to know how hard and demanding growing a top shelf crop can actually be; and brother, I mean demanding. If you look on the internet or U-Tube there are countless growers that do it organically and do it right. They are meticulous on growing the ganja they would want for themselves. Since everything in this industry is secret there is no way to tell what growers supply to what Co-Op.

Without knowing where the herb came from, you really don't know how it was grown. Wherever there is money involved, you can bet your life there are unscrupulous people trying to take advantage of the unknowing. If one of your plants gets the mold, you will quarantine the sickly plant or even trash it if there is any doubt at all. You would never ingest a plant with questionable concerns about your personal safety; can you say that about other growers? There are tales about growers using growth hormones to increase yield and the all mighty profit margin; a substance band for all consumable products but still legal to sell to use on your boxwood or bougainvillea plants. If your garden gets an attack from a hungry swarm of insects, you will do all you can to correct the problem organically. This is a much more time consuming method but it's the better and safer way.

A grower with concerns of profit over safety will likely take the easy way out and use the poison to save time, money and his beloved profit.

I guess the bottom line is; how was it grown? When you've grown it on your own, there is never a question, concern or doubt; you know it's done the correct and safest way. Not only will it give you a since of pride on your finished product, it will give you piece of mind on every medication. With all that said, not only will you learn to grow the finest ganja possible, you may just have a whole lot of fun doing it. If you like to grow vegetables, fruit trees, orchids or roses, I'm willing to bet you will find cannabis cultivation much more entertaining in multiple ways.

Not only will you know how your meds were grown; not only will you find entertainment in your endeavor; you're hard, but enjoyable work will save you two hundred dollars and more every single month on your med bill. This is why I say if you have the ware with all, growing your own cannabis is not only rewarding; it's rewarding.

There are some things about growing I think are well worth mentioning. Before you start anything check out the web or published books for and endless supply of information. Like most everything, there is more than one way to skin a cat and growing ganja is certainly one of them. You will find one guy saying this is the way to do it and another guy doing it a totally different way. One grower will say pick off the dying leaves because they are pulling strength from the plant while another swears the buds are pulling stored reserves from the leaves. One grower swears by one recipe on soil mix while the other has a completely different mix. One guy likes nutrient A while the other likes B. One person thinks watering from the top is best, and yes, the other thinks the bottom watering works best. What works for one may not work as good for the other so you should do a little research and try each way until a particular system works best for you and the environment you're working in. Personally I leave the leaves on until they are quite dead with no more reserves to pull from. I also like the bottom watering. If you fill a saucer the soil will absorb the water and it will peculate up. I think the watering on the bottom attracts the roots down. I know that because when you water from a saucer the roots will come out of the drain hole chasing water. They don't do that when I water from the top. Once the roots come out about a half inch you automatically know without guesswork it's time for a larger pot.

Even though there are different ways to do some things, other things require strict discipline and ridged requirements. One thing you never want to do is reinvent the wheel and make the same mistakes others have already made. Experience usually shows the way and long time growers have learned the right and wrong way to do things. Light for instance. If your grow room is under lit, the ladies will be weak and skinny with a small yield; however, over lit rooms will result in too much heat and wasted electricity. Another problem is too much light and heat can actually slow down photosynthesis unless CO_2 is entered into the equation. Carbon dioxide will certainly increase the growth rate of a plant considering it's what it lives on; and in return, our friend the plants give off oxygen we need to live. Seems like a pretty good system to me.

Ventilation and air circulation is just as important as light. Without air movement the natural CO_2 in the air, about 350 parts per million, won't flow around the leaves giving good breathing to the plant. The air flow is also for bending and wiggling the stem and branches to increase strength and thickness. Grow boxes need two or more fans depending on the size of the room. One set of fans removes the heat from the light and the humidity from plants and soil via 4 or 6 inch ducting. Another set of fans is the oscillating type placed on the wall for circulation of air contained inside the box. Here again, there is all sorts of calculators on the web. They have calculators for electric bills, calculators on what size light you need for a particular sized room, calculators on what size fan you need and on and on it goes. If you're going to build, build right so your garden will show the right results.

A grow box can be anything from the simple to the sublime. Since pot likes to grow in the upper seventy degrees range with humidity of forty to sixty percent, serious growers will bow to their ladies every need. They will incorporate air conditioning units in the summer and trade them out for heaters in the winter. They will add humidifiers in dry weather and dehumidifiers in moist weather. They will check religiously the Ph of the soil and adjust its alkaline or acidic depending on its needs. They will add CO_2 at various times with the help of a control panel and some go all the way with various types of fast growing hydroponic systems.

Everything just mentioned will certainly add speed to the growth and weight to the yield; but, it will also require much more time, effort and experience; not to mention a much heftier dollar investment in your medical garden. All this information is readily available, but unless you're extraordinary I would suggest starting out slowly and building your garden with understanding and experience; not on your well intended hopes and wishes.

Chapter Eleven: *My thoughts,*

reflections and opinions.

    I guess it's time for my own opinions after using for a little over two years. There certainly are a lot of unanswered questions with regards to medical marijuana. Questions like: 1) should it be legal for anyone to use? 2) Is an inebriant really able to be of medical use? 3) Will the potency remain as intense as the first time I used it or will I get used to it over time? 4) Are the negatives worth the positives? 5) Will I become addicted to it? 6) Is legalized cannabis a viable medicine or just a conceived scam to get stoned legally? 7) Is an industry so secret and hush, hush able to provide safe, well grown ganja to its patients? 8)Will it make me want stronger drugs?

    All of these seem to be very good questions and like most good questions different people will have different answers. I can only answerer these questions as how they regard to me. You will get answers saying pot is the end all of cure alls while others believe it to be the plant of the Devil himself. I've heard of some people believing no medicine should ever be used because faith in the All Mighty is the only medicine man or woman ever needs.

Maybe it comes down to different strokes for different folks. But whatever it comes down too, you can bet there will be controversy and misunderstanding from one belief to another.

Should grass be legal to use by anyone and everyone? I've thought about this long and hard with different opinions at different times. This high strength marijuana is definitely not for kids. Do I want some Newbie out at a bar drinking and smoking the strong stuff? Not in this millennium I don't. Young kids seem to think they're invincible and can not only do, but can get away with anything; that is until they lose control of the car and destroy themselves and worse; some unknowing poor soul just trying to go home from work.

Kids just don't seem to think at times. They think they're thinking, but actually they're just thinking they can get away with it. They never think about what happens when they don't. I remember once in my early twenties a few buddies were coming home from the Lake Elsinore in two different cars. My friend that killed the rat was driving his '70 Cuda and I was in my '55 T-Bird hauling butt down the I-15 Freeway at 70 miles an hour. Since one car had the cold Pepsi's and one car had the hot doobies, we simply brought the cars within two feet of each other and nonchalantly passed the sodas over and the joints back. Since those were the days before radial tires, the bias type would track on every groove of the road making the car swerve from side to side. A kid doesn't think about that; he wants a cold pop and a hot doobie; pulling off the highway and wasting time wouldn't even have been considered. I'm not blaming it all on ganja. If we were beer drinkers I'm sure it would have been bottles that were passed over. I wouldn't admit it in writing, and I'm very sorry to admit, but I've done much dumber thing than that.

I'm to the opinion the use of marijuana should only be used by a person who has their work ethics set in stone, their goals and dreams already in the planning, their moral compass pointing due North and the ability to feel comfortable in their own skin without worry of other peoples opinions. Without these personal traits ganja might have a way of turning you into a dreamer and not a doer. A good Indica has a way of making you lazy and if you can't control your own emotions then Pot may be a hindrance to you over a help.

If I had a choice of legal marijuana or alcohol, now, I would have to say marijuana by tenfold. I know, three years ago I would have never even considered such an option; and that's why I've thought long and hard on the subject. I'm not one for trying to take away a person's choice or their rights but alcohol is a big enough problem for the nation. I'm sure with so many unanchored people a legalized marijuana would probably add to the problem; although, that's only my opinion. Another thing, do you take something away from the 90 percent just because 10 percent of the people can't handle it? A friend of mine that hasn't partaken in any drink or smoke for thirty years used to really down the booze in his younger years. I mean, he guzzled it. He never smoked tobacco but he did his fair share of pot smoking at the same time. While I like the relaxing mellowness of ganja, he preferred being drunk to that of being stoned. Even in the days of my scotch drinking I never liked being drunk. A warm relaxing buzz was looked forward too, but the double vision, the slurring words, the staggering and the much hated bed spins are bad enough, but the hangovers were never worth it. When I was young I could get rid of a Hanover by the end of the next day; now it takes me a week from Tuesday.

With booze you can drink yourself unconscious up to the point of dying. I don't think I can vaporize myself unconscious and I know I can't kill myself with an overdose. I have never forgotten what happened the night before or staggered down the hall when I walked off to bed. I have never seen double or woken with a killer hangover; or any hangover at all for that matter. It seems to me, with marijuana, you get to a certain point and you go no further. To me five hits may get you very high while ten hits are nowhere near double your high. If you're skunk drunk on five shots, after ten you'd be out cold on the floor wallowing in your own vomit. This never happens with herb.

These are the reasons why I chose Herb over alcohol. But, like everything, it's not to say cannabis is without its faults. I never drive when medicated not only because it's against the law, but I just don't feel comfortable doing it. I've worked too hard for what I have and I sure don't want to give it up in a lousy lawsuit; however, I know many people that do in regards to both drinking and medicating. One is the guy that kicked the quarter like a hacky sack and caught it in air; the guy that pimps the herb. I'm not too sure he couldn't drive was well as some and better than most. It would be interesting to have one of those police driving test with a real drinking man against a long time medical user. Let them drive through the course sober and then get them ripped and have them do it again. I'm not so sure the Pimp would do any worse. If I remember right, back in the day after we downed a few bowls we would have some pretty darn good ping pong games which takes quite a bit of eye-hand coordination. I mean, we weren't as good as Forest Gump, but we would get some hot rallies going out in my friend's garage late on Saturday night.

Speaking of eye-hand coordination while under the influence; one day we probably had a little more than normal before our game. I was odd man out so I watched two friends battle out the first game. About half way through one friend stopped playing and looked at his opponent with shock on his face. After a minute of staring he looked around the workbench behind him and picked up a 12 inch screwdriver. With one might heave he tossed the projectile, what looked to be, right at my other friend. Actually, it missed him by a good five feet, but it didn't miss the rat crawling up one of the wood studs. I'm telling you the screwdriver hit that sucker dead center and pinned him on the two by four stud without the vermin moving a muscle; dead on contact. I imagine you could understand what three loaded kids looked like whooping and hollering and running around in circles in victory over the beast. It was such a prize the mummified rat was still stuck up there three months later. It was proof to everyone that didn't believe us.

The next question asked is an inebriant viable for medical use. Since I have already discussed what it does for me, I can only say what others have told me and what testimonials I've seen on TV and the Web. If something helps a person to stay away from hanging on to everyday's individual minutes with their fingernails, to them it is very viable. If something helps a person find comfort for just a few hours a day; to them it's very viable. If something helps keep a person's head out of the toilet; to them it's very viable.

The next question is will I get used to herb or will it always be as intense. This is a different answerer than I expected. After a few years of medicating I'm much closer to understanding what the guy meant when he said, "I pimp the medicine and don't let the medicine pimp me." I haven't used near as long as he has but I do know the high is not near as intense as it was at first. I liken it to making love. It seems like the first few times were much better but you still never get tired of it. Herb doesn't get you as stoned, but it still does what it always did. Your thought process while medicated is not so unsure on what's happening around you; especially with Sativa. A good strain seems to channel your thoughts while with the Indica it doesn't matter. That's for nap and bedtime. You don't have to think then.

Are the negatives worth the positives? You know, when I say this I really mean it; I haven't found too many negative's in marijuana. The price is one very big negative, but what's the price for deep sound sleep? Having to be secret and hush, hush about growing is a big negative, but being able to save hundreds a month is no negative. Having to spend so much time and effort in farming can be a negative, but what you get out of watching and enjoying a crop grow into the ganja you want is nowhere close to being a negative. Growing a small yield is a negative, but learning how to increase yield or learning anything is a great positive. Doing something you spent your whole life talking against and keeping that something away from your kids is a great big negative…I don't think there is a positive in that one.

Will I become addicted to marijuana? Again, I'm only speaking for me; although, I have read a few studies where they say no. I say the same thing. There has been a time I went on vacation and had to leave the weed at home for two weeks. Although I missed the sleep, I never thought once about it. With cigarettes I would have spent every single minute of the trip thinking about smoking. There has been a time when I was out of herb but didn't want to, or couldn't afford to, take a hundred bucks out of the budget for medicine. I didn't sleep well, but I was nowhere near the wanting I'd previously known from other addictions.

Now it's down to the last two questions. Is medical marijuana a scam, and how can a secret industry supply safe, consistent and reliable medicine to the unknowing patient? The answer is maybe it can and maybe it can't; maybe it can sometimes but I highly doubt it can all the time. I might have to be a little careful with this one. Many words could be written on this subject and there would probably be many facts to support both sides. As far as it being a scam, I'm sorry to say, I think a bigger portion than should be is definitely bogus. It allows some people a legal way to party with ganja with no medical value needed or wanted. There are others, I imagine, that really think they need the herb but are just using its psychoactive properties to run away from the real problem; as does some alcoholics. Although, in most circles, alcohol is a deadly disease and has a much more addictive personality than marijuana ever thought of having. The way I look at it is along the lines of; Herb only likes you no matter how much you love it, while you may like alcohol but the booze can love you so much it doesn't want to ever let you go. Again, this is only my opinion and I'm certainly not one to tell a responsible person what to do or in what to believe. Maybe the matter should be left up to the individual states and how their societies vote on the matter. Enough of politics. (Yuck)

When it comes to a secret industry I know for a fact there are some very responsible growers that anyone would have a difficult time reproducing the same results; be it quality of the meds or the meticulous method in which it is organically grown. There are no doubts about the very good and responsible growers bringing a safe and primo product to the market. The only problem is; how do you know for certain a good grower is supplying the meds? A person may tell you it's grown in the strictest of methods, but again, can you believe it? There is also the fact that the older you get the fewer people you trust. Time tells you in no certain way people will take shortcuts when able, take the easy way out more times than not, and think of their profits over the well being of someone they will never know or even meet. The best way to know just how a crop was treated is to grow it yourself.

Of course that may not be an option, but if it is, you have to understand it is no simple task to be a good marijuana farmer. When I first heard a patient was allowed to have twelve plants I thought it was way in excess; and it might be if you could grow unrestricted under the natural sun. However, 99 percent of the people are not able to grow outside; mostly because of security concerns. When you first start out you may get a yield of four wet ounces that dry down to an ounce. If you smoked a quarter of an ounce a week you would consume in one month what took five or six months to grow. At that rate you can keep even but if you use a little more you will be back at the Co-Op reaching for a hard earned hundred bucks; if you lose a crop you will be buying for six months. Not good in any growers book.

The only way to prevent disaster is through knowledge and experience. Only time can give you experience, but there is a wealth of information to increase your knowledge. When you seek information be very sure to pay close attention to the optimal. In other words, to be a successful grower you must and need to increase your yield. Remember to try and not reinvent the wheel. Over time growers have learned what the optimal is and to increase yield you must bow to the ladies optimal. For cannabis foliage to prosper and for maximum photosynthesis the plant prefers the temperature to be in the mid to upper seventies. For the roots to absorb the proper level of nutrients they like the temp to be in the upper sixties.

Since optimal increases yield it can't be emphasized enough how important it is to find ways to reach the optimum. If you're growing in your garage in winter and the lights bring the temp up to a warm eighty degrees, the moment the lights go out the temp could drop down to a very chilly freezing;

which of course, is nowhere near to optimal. With extremes like that the chances of losing your entire crop is indeed intensified. And, of course, in the summer when the ambient temperature is one hundred the light can add twenty degrees and more. Now you're on the other end of the spectrum where the heat will shut a plant down.

I'm lucky I live in So Cal where the weather is never extreme for more than a few days at a time. I worry much more in regards to the heat in August over the cold in February. Since I don't have either a heater or an air conditioner for my two small grow rooms, I try to make the light work for me. In the heat of the summer and the cold of winter I burn the lights at night. In the winter the air is cold and the plants love the warm lights. In the summer nights are cooler preventing overheating in the daytime hours where no amount of ventilation will bring down the heat. On very hot spells I may bring the watts down from 1000 to 600 and even from 600 to 400 for very short spells of time. Any lower light will result in the plants stressing and possibly floundering no matter how short the time period.

In spring and fall I can burn the lights during the hours that suit me best; although, when your lights run 18 hours and 12 hours a day you can pretty well set your timers to work with your own schedule. One thing you cannot do under any circumstance when the plants are flowering is interrupt their 12 hours of darkness. They need twelve hours of pure darkness and nothing less. It's been said even a bight full moon can stress the plant out of flowering or into hermaphrodite. They say if you can't work the 12 hour light into your schedule, a green light in your flowering room has no effect on them. Remember, optimum for this particularly fussy plant is the right light, ventilation, water, nutrients, temperature, humidity, and Ph; not necessarily in that order, but one can be just as deadly or just as helpful as the other. But when these elements are working together in harmony, the results can be astonishing.

Diligence, knowledge and tenacity are the only things that will dramatically increase your yield. If you're going to spend time and money growing a plant, you might as well go the few extra steps and grow it right. I'm not saying you'll get 500 grams out of every square meter like the brochures say; I know I sure haven't. But that's not to say with more experience and knowledge it won't happen. As my knowledge grows, so does my yield. My first couple of plants grown under 100% artificial light was a mere ounce of dried weight per bush. It was a mile away from 500 grams stated, but it was still enough to keep me in herb.

As I kept harvesting the yields kept growing. First it was one and a half oz; then two and then two and a half; then three, and now I am up to four and more ounces per plant. By the looks of some of the ladies coming due, I think I'll be breaking my own records every time I harvest. Since I try to stagger the time of my plants harvest, my goal is to have a plant ready to crop every three to four weeks. You can quickly see four ounces or more of meds per month is way more herb than I need. I believe if I can do it pretty much anyone can do it; especially people with green thumbs and able to understand the ways of the species they nurture.

This little problem we all want sometimes leads to another dilemma; what to do with all the extra ganja? I don't know what other states are but California allows a patient to keep up to eight ounces of buds. Like all parts of the law this too is ambiguous. One part of the law says you can have six mature plants and six immature at any one time; however, if you harvested just one plant that gave you 500 grams you would be out of compliance by over nine ounces. How's that supposed to work? I guess the Senate in there wise and wondrous ways realized most people can't get a harvest near that large by growing indoors; again, which most growers are forced to do. But what if you are a great grower and realize a crop every bit as large?

Well, one way, and the worst way, is to compost the overage. Believe me; it hurts just to type the sentence. After such painstaking work and nurturing your plants so carefully it's almost sacrilege to destroy nine ounces of primo bud; no, on second thought, it is very definitely sacrilege. Another option is to hide it where no one can find it; but you'd still be breaking the law.

In California, by the law, a Co-Op has to be non-profit in all respects and aspects. The law says you can volunteer time, barter and even work for the industry if you take a reasonable amount to run the business or do the job. Boy, that word "reasonable" sure is a scary term. What does it even mean? Who knows? What it means to me is if I see I might have a little extra herb that will put me over my allotted amount of eight ounces, I certainly want to visit one of my friendly neighborhood Co-Ops to see if they're in need of some buds over the option of having my tears raining rivers in the compost bin.

Beware of first trying out this step. Most Co-Ops will tell you they get their weed form special members or from growers up in Humboldt; and they're certainly not lying. But what they are saying between the lines is; "I have to have quality meds to stay in business and quality meds is something most people can't come close to achieving on a regular basis." And you know, that's fine, too. You'd do the exact same thing if you were in his shoes. Chances are if you take the walk into medical marijuana you will be buying and evaluating the effects on you long before you will be growing. During this time try and make friends with your Co-Op. Study different strains and carry a conversation that will subtly let them know your knowledge of medical cannabis is more than just buying pot. As you make purchases of different strains you will fast become aware of how heavy, thick, dense and fragrant each bud is. There is absolutely no leaves or major stems what-so-ever; just pure thick and sticky buds. Unless you're really good, the buds on your first harvest will look nothing like the store bought type. They will probably be loose, leafy, thin and green. The ganja may give pretty good effects but the taste, smell and smoke ability will leave a lot to be desired; and chances are your bud is like it is because you missed a very important step.

Five or six months of very slow growing and flowering can be ruined if curing isn't done properly. It won't take you long to realize curing is every bit, if not more important, than growing. In a lot of ways it's much harder to achieve. After months of anticipation you are egar to see the results of your hard and tedious labors. The tendency by new growers is to force dry a bud in the oven or microwave and give it a try. When you're totally disappointed in the product don't blame it on the weed; blame it on the cure. The secret to curing is slow, slow, slow, slow, slow. Should I say it again to make it clear? The secret is slow, slow, slow. I had to find that out by hard experience between a summer crop and a winter crop.

In summer you can hang a plant to dry in the garage and it will be ready for the curing jar in three days if you don't regulate the drying; another three or four days in the jar and it will be about as dry as you want it. Now let's take a look at the winter harvest. At sixty degrees it won't dry in two days, it takes two weeks or more; yep, and another week or more in the jar. With this slow drying time you will notice the bud has lost its green and became a little on the brown side. This is good in all respects. The bud has dissipated the chlorophyll and pulled down into a thick, dense and sticky bud. If you crack open a jar of summertime quick-dry harvest and compare the fragrance and looks with a slow dry winter harvest the differences will become painfully clear; fast dry is poor while slow dry is primo.

This is why most Co-Ops don't want to mess with a novice grower. To be good it takes consistency in cloning, veging, flowering, curing; and every person in the industry knows it. But believe me, good bud is something everyone is interested in; the question is who will buy it legally? This is where a little effort on your part will come in handy. If you take a good quality bud to an owner and let him try it out, if it's as good as you think it is; then so will he. It's your job to get him to believe in your abilities as a grower and to build trust so in the event of an overage he'll be more than happy to take your few ounces of surplus without fear.

Since THC doesn't like heat or light I have my own way of storing excess. I usually keep about a week's worth in my med box and I keep three to four weeks in a sealed jar kept in a cool dark part of the house ready for immediate use. Anything more and I vacuum seal two ounces per bag and keep the entire vacuum sealed bag in a jar placed in the bottom corner of the Frigidaire. I'm told it will keep in there until man walks on Mars. If I'm adding to the excess, which doesn't happen with every harvest, I take a jar from the frig and barter with the Co-Op. Since I'm not into growing for money over what I save, all I want is to cover the electric bill and nutrients if I can. There is times when I'll take half the price the Co-Op is willing to pay if they pass the saving on to their needy customers. This seems to work out for all concerned with truth filled "thank yous" and "you're welcome" all around.

I guess this is where I am in my walk into medical marijuana. I must say it's been a very interesting experience. Even though I've learned a powerful lot about cannabis, I know with everything I've learned it only adds to the questions I've been trying to find answers to. I guess that old adage stands true: "the more you learn clarifies how much you really don't know."

Yes, I've learned a lot and I hope to keep on learning. I have to tell you there were things that really surprised me in regards to medical marijuana. I guess the biggest surprise is how something voted by the people to be legal can be so damn shady. I guess it's the nature of the beast; but still, shouldn't a legal substance be grown, transported to Co-Ops and sold to patients without the stigma of being under worldly or downright criminal? Shouldn't a person be able to grow without fear of the police knocking on the door or some dick head thief breaking into your home and possibly doing bodily harm for a plant not unlike corn, orchids, roses and tomatoes?

But when I really think about it, it's not at all hard to understand it. Only a couple of years ago

I was in the same frame of mind and couldn't help thinking about how I was so against it in any form and how I always tried to keep my kids away from it and the other fifty youth kicking party drugs. I remember thinking about it deeply one night. My thoughts took me to a time my son was five or six. Since he's almost got his hands on forty you can see how far my mind took me back. If I remember right it was around Christmas or New Years when my wife and I and another couple want a little party bag to ring in the New Year. Well, usually my wife's brother could get whatever we wanted; but he was out of town and unavailable. Now, this was at a time when they figured out how to test for marijuana in the system; this is also the time they began drug and random drug testing.

For this reason I wasn't real keen on the use of marijuana like I was a year or two before. My career was starting to go and a lousy high wasn't even close to trading your job for; so really, at the time I was thinking hard about staying away from it. It was on that night way back when that I decided to stay away from weed and I stayed away for the better part of thirty-five years.

Since my brother-in-law was unavailable, my wife got the address where I could go grab a quick ounce and be back before our friends arrived. Since my wife and I both had things to do, I grabbed the boy and my daughter went with her Mom. When I got to the guy house it was 5:30, pitch dark, and the street had no lights. I drove into the driveway and told my son to wait in the car. The only light to the door was the residual light from the cars headlights and I'm telling you a very strange feeling came over me. As I stood on the porch I looked back at my son. Since it was the days before child car seats, he was standing in the seat looking at me with his patented cute kid face.

When Iknocked on the door I kept looking at the child as the strange feeling just kept getting worse and worse. I finally asked myself what the hell I was doing at a home of some unknown person trying to pick up a totally illegal drug with my own boy in the car. In that one split second of time I knew something was really screwed up and I want out of the situation as fast as I could get away. About that time the door opened by a man right out of the Harley Davidson book of motorcycles and beer drinking brawls. He had a big thick beard and his long hair was held in place with a Harley bandana. He had the bike boots, the Quick Silver T-shirt and a pair of dirty Levi's with more holes in them than material. In a gruff voice he asked, "Yeah, what do you want?"

I wanted out of there as fast as I could get so I just answered, "You don't look like Mr. Gordon. They told me to go to 619 Duel Street."

The guy just sneered at me and growled, "Duel is the next street over," and then he slammed the door in my face. I wanted out fast and I just got what I wanted. When I got home I thought I might get some static when I told wifey I didn't even ask him and I wasn't sure if I would ever smoke again. I was shocked when she left the kitchen saying, "Maybe it's for the better." Most of the time we never agreed on anything much less having us agreeing on something. I didn't realize it at the time but this is around the time she really started drinking. I found out she had quite a drinking problem before I met her, but somehow she got the problem under control and I was never even aware of it for the first two years of marriage. Looking back I sure wish she had told me about her problem. It would have been no trouble for me to keep beer and alcohol out of the house and away from her temptation since it was no big deal to me. This is another thing you might want to be aware of in the land of medical marijuana; in a medicated state your mind has a tendency to run wild thinking about things far into your past. Not only will you think of things you thought you had forgotten all about, it will make you analyze your mistakes and second guess yourself on life changing problems and if they could have been avoided with a little caution. You know the past can't be changed but it sure doesn't stop your mind from wondering "what if".

Another thing about the modern cannabis that surprised me was the different types of "high" that can be reached. It's amazing to me how a different strain can be so totally different from the next. I always try to see what's new from the breeders, but I have my two or three favorites and it will take a lot to steal me away from White Widow and Medijuana. For me the Widow is just such a beautifully clear high compared to any other I've tried. I know if you never used you might not understand what a "clear" high means; and I'm thinking unless you know what I'm talking about you'll never know what I'm talking about; it's that complicated. It's a high that doesn't fight itself by clouding thoughts and new ideas. It's just a beautifully clear head high is all I can say.

Medijuana, on the other hand, is kick butt medicine made for sleep and not much more than sleep. Unlike the clean and clear Widow's high, Medi-girl will cloud your thoughts with dreams and fantasies. It will take you out of your time zone and drop you wherever she thinks fit. Most of the time Medi is a warm and relaxing ride with the only goal

a soft bed and a restful night's sleep. Oh, what
sweet words for an insomniac.

My third strain I like a lot is a plant simply
called Ice. It's another medical strength strain and
Cannabis Cup winner besides. An original strain
like this had to be crossed with Afghan, Northern
Lights, Skunk and Shiva. I like Ice for its cool
Vape, high THC content and the way it grows short
but harvests big; getting back to the yield, you
know. Ice's buds are intensely coated with
beautiful white crystals giving it a sweet taste and a
very relaxing but extremely heavy stone.

This is an example of what good cannabis
breeding has come to. That's why I said earlier
breeding should be left to the big boys. Having a
limit of only six veging plants a patient could never
cross breed so many strains to come up with a cup
winner. Let them do it so you can enjoy the labors
of their work and not waste time hoping one of your
crosses will turn into killer herb.

These are my three favorites but I haven't
come close to trying even half the strains available;
and I'm sure I never will. Now I'm to the point of
knowing what I like and don't like. I've had strains
that left me so nervous and fidgety I couldn't relax
with the help of two beautiful masseuses pressing
palms against my aching body. Being very un-

comfortable is going against the purpose of trying to be comfortable. Other strains have left me moody while another may give me the blues; one will make me giggly while the other will make me quiet; one will make me hungry with the munchies and another won't. It all depends on who you are and what it is. One thing's for sure, if it's not right for you there are many more varieties out there with probably more than one bred to your perfect match.

Obviously, one of the big surprises of medical marijuana was the price. I tell you I almost fainted dead away when Mr. Mohawk told me it was a hundred bucks for a quarter of an ounce; not a hundred bucks for a full ounce. Weed might be very difficult to grow under artificial conditions, but I know for a fact it grows like a weed outdoors. I don't know if you've ever driven through Castroville when the artichokes were in flower, but the fields go on and on and on for as far as the eye can see. If one single field was replace with a good Sativa or Indica the price would freefall down to mere dollars an ounce; a far piece from a Ben Franklin for a quarter oz. But it is what it is so growing your own is way more fun and far less expensive.

Another thing that really surprised me in this industry is how many young people are patients. When I go over to Kaiser Permanente for my epidural or yearly check up, most of the people I see are gray haired and walking with a cane. It's just the opposite in medical marijuana Co-Ops. Most of the people are young and dumb and not so many are gray and wise. This small fact may tell you something about the medical marijuana system; I'm not saying, I'm just saying.

I can't figure out how so many young people get away with being a marijuana patient without getting fired. When I was working there was drug testing and random drug testing. I'm willing to bet not one of my employers would even half way care if I was a marijuana patient. If I failed the test, I'd be asked to not let the door hit me in the ass on the way out. These young kids have to be working to afford a hundred bucks a quarter; I mean, after all, you can get street weed for much cheaper than Co-Op meds. I wondered if their employer's were very understanding or if I was the only one called in for random testing.

I did learn how some pass the drug test when I sold my '50 Pontiac to a guy that sent it down to Australia. To hear the buyer tell it he just closed down a business he made quite a bit of money from; he closed it down because the DEA gave him a cease and desist or they would raid his place and take him to court. I don't know how much the guy made off the business, but the way he was hinting about it was close to a million. He seemed happy with it and didn't want to take on the DEA even though he was "almost" sure he would win.

His little invention was quite unique and one I never heard of. It was a belt you wore under your pants and skivvies with a rubber reservoir filled with phony urine. The bag nestles in your groin for warmth and can be whipped out your pants as though you were really peeing. I got to say its very cleaver but you'd have to have some mighty big balls to wear a bag of synthetic urine into a drug test. He said the phony urine would fool any lab.

I guess the hardest things that took me by surprise was the level of knowledge and experience it takes to produce a perpetual growing garden high in quality along with high producing yields. I certainly wish I would have thought it out a little better before I attacked the gardening portion of the equation. My big mistake was not listening to men like Ed Rosenthal or Jorge Cervantes who trail blazed the process decades before my arrival on scene. Their videos are all over U-Tube to be watched and books at the store to be studied. When men of experience give you the optimal parameters on various stages of growing it behooves anyone to lend them your ear. They know what they're doing and what they do will work for you as well. Their knowledge is sure helping me to produce a fine garden I'm proud of in every way. It's too bad that something you're so proud of has to be kept top secret. In my opinion this part of the equation just doesn't add up; but it is what it is.

The big question; will cannabis push me to stronger and harder drugs. It is a very good question and one that truly bothered me when I first started medicating. You know I can only speak for myself, but I can truthfully say I have never once thought of taking a harder drug or even wandering what they were like. All I was looking for was some sleep and with medical cannabis I have found what I was looking for. There is no need to look farther.

Chapter Twelve: *Closing thoughts.*

Most of the people I know don't smoke or drink. Therefore my close friends who know I medicate have all asked the same question; "has the medical marijuana helped you?" It's the best question you could ask and it will take a little explaining.

Fist I have to emphatically say I would much rather lose the numbness and tingling in my arms and hands than to use medical cannabis in any way, shape or form. Unfortunately for me the pain management doctors and surgeons don't seem to think a risky operation is worth it at this time. When they tell me they can't fix me right now I always have to wonder if they could fix me if I was a twenty-three year old fire-throwing pitcher for the Los Angeles Dodgers. I wonder. On the other hand I'm not sure I want to go through having my neck opened, spine removed and replaced for a 20 percent chance it will work. I don't mind being called chicken. If I knew the 20 percent would be successful I would grab it in a New York second; it's the eighty percent that puts the lump in the throat and the weakness in the knees. When it gets to 50 /50 get the table ready. I'm on the way.

I say this for a very simple reason. When a man uses and relies on his hands his whole life, it's more than depressing when the uses of one's hands are taken away. It's hard to think about the days when you could work on your hot rods all day long and not give it a single thought except how nice the bed will feel. The thought of painting houses, building cabinets, tiling floors, replacing windows, typing sales orders all day, or hand sanding a chest for hours on end seems so impossible to achieve but remembered when it was looked forward too with enthusiasm and reverence. I don't know how others would handle it, but I thought if a man didn't have his hands, he couldn't call himself a man; when a person couldn't do what he loved to do, it's easy to manifest the situation into not having a reason. When things get so low from being bone tired or racked with pain the thought of having no reason seems to be intensified by a thousand. It's even worse when you know there's no such thing as how nice the bed will feel. It can never feel nice when the night is not your friend.

It got to the point I didn't like much of anything. Not only did I not like it, I was getting pretty lousy at doing anything. It was almost like one of those old 1930's movies when somebody slowly worked themselves to a miserable death. I never really believed it until I started to feel like it.

Every little chore was a mental fight to complete; just the opposite of how I used to be. I would never put anything off and look forward to the next challenge with gusto; not any more, I don't. I knew it very clearly back in 2009 in the depths of this miserable recession when things were far from looking good at any angle of my life. Like most businesses, the company I worked for found things quite tight due to the lousy California economy. With that came rumors of layoffs. I hate to admit it, but I was hopping one of the layoffs would be me. It just seemed I couldn't do, or even enjoy, my job like I used to do. After leaving the regular job I worked weeknights and every weekend for almost a year. I had just finished very hard work completely redoing the inside of my home; and I mean everything from the kitchen, bathroom, copper plumbing, three-wire electric, floors, carpet and new windows. I felt like I was in one of those old-time movies; you know the guy that's works so hard he spent his last reserves. I was having a hard time making it through the day and I knew I wasn't giving my employer my full day's best. When you're not at your best, and you know you're not at your best, it takes all the dreadful and depressing thoughts and intensifies them even more. When all these things start to load on you, it becomes hard to look forward to tomorrow.

I was actual happy when I got laid off. I figured if I could just relax for a month or so to chill and recuperate, I could get back to my same old self. I figured I could reenergize and get back to the excitement of a new job. My plan didn't work in several ways. First, after three months I wasn't feeling any better; I was feeling worse and sleeping even less. Not only was I feeling worse in my health, being home all the time was next to being in prison. Being an outside salesman most of my life, I missed seeing my customers and meeting new people every day. But I also knew to the bottom of my heart it was easy for me to understand I just didn't have it anymore. Something was missing and every single minute of every single day I longed for it back. After three months of supposedly recouping, I wasn't sleeping, relaxing or feeling any better on any level.

The first way my plan didn't work was I didn't get any better; I actually got worse. The second way it didn't work took me by total surprise. Most of the time during my layoff I was actively seeking employment. I found out in the last ten years the job hunt market had changed dramatically. It used to be a company needing to hire would simply advertize in the local newspaper for applicants and a person could polish up the old resume and drop it off at the address given.

Sometimes you could get a quick interview on the spot and that's where I've excelled my whole life long. When I went into an interview I was so arrogantly cocky I expected to get whatever job was available whether I had experience in the field or not. I would do my very best to make the interviewer believe I would make them proud of their decision to take me on. I made them believe I could learn any job and work harder than anyone else. I would sit there and look them in the eye when I told them and, what's more, I believed every single word of it. I truly was so arrogant and cocky I believed if they didn't hire me it was for the best because somebody that dumb couldn't be working for a very good company. I guess it was for that reason I was never unemployed for long and I didn't think anything had changed.

Oh, but a lot changed. Now the newspaper was replaced with Monster and other web job finders. Now the dropping off of your resume was replaced with email. Now, instead of looking them in the eye as you told them about yourself, they get their information solely from the resume; and in an employer's market they can be very picky when it comes to what they want. Do you speak two languages; do you have a degree in this field; are you willing to take a greater salary and smaller benefits. Wow, what a change. When you're twenty-five you work for money; when 62 you work for bennies. I mean, come on. How are you supposed to BS your way into a job if you can't look then in the eye?

Yeah, it was another sobering fact that hit me hard, and with everything else, I was really nearing my whit's end. I was not only going downhill physically, the mental avalanche might seem to be taking me down even faster. At the time I didn't know what to do or where to begin even if I knew what to do. It was one of the only times in my life I was unsure, scared and all alone. It was a place I did not like being.

Like it or not, I was there and I would spend a week there every single day of my life. I knew I could never give a man an honest day's work in the condition I was in so, against my own will, I was forced to think about early retirement. I was on Cobra and since it was only months away from my 62nd birthday I thought I might be able to inch it out until then. I'm happy to say I think with my past practices I did it right. My house is paid for and I carry no debt in any way, so it doesn't take much for me to survive. I have to say I was very lucky by getting out of the dot com bubble as well as the real-estate bubble. When you live long enough you are able to see these bubbles and fads much clearer than when you're young and dumb.

I remember in March of 2007 I was having morning coffee when a real estate lady put up a for sale sign on the house across the street. When I went to talk to her she told me the house was listed at 490 thousand dollars, I almost dropped my coffee cup. Although I bought my house thirty-six years ago it only cost me $23,500. At the time I was making 18 grand a year plus company car and a possible thousand dollar a year bonus. I can remember sweating about being able to meet the $230 mortgage when my rent was $70 a month and sometimes I had trouble coming up with that payment. Now, if you think about it, my home cost me a few thousand dollars more than I made in a year. When I retired I made 70 thousand a year; 490 thousand isn't a few thousand dollars more than I make a year; it's almost five times my yearly salary. Hell, I don't think I could afford my own house. Obviously something has gone haywire with housing and I knew it right after my conversation with the real estate lady. I immediately went in and switched my 401K from stocks to bonds, turned most of my portfolio into cash and I liquidated all my real estate holdings. At first I thought I really screwed up because the stock market and real estate just kept going up; that is until October when the bottom literally fell out of both markets; at least the biggest drop in my lifetime. Man, running from those markets was the smartest thing I did in my entire life; it enabled me to retire with my home paid and my mailbox full of junk but with no bills to be found. Retirement came about five years early and I'm not near where I dreamed retirement would take me, but it's enough to get by and I'm thankful for that.

My advice to young people; unless you have a bank full of money, you better plan on having your house paid for by the time you reach retirement; that means you cannot have more than a fifteen year note when your 50. At that time it would be stupid to take out a thirty year note unless you think you can work till your eighty. Take the advice of someone who's been there and done that; pay your house off and get rid of all your bills; then money, one of the most stressful things a person has to contend with, will never have to be contended with. Not only that, it will increase your buying power by three or four times. That's like getting a raise in pay. So what if you have to sweat for awhile to pay the mortgage? Time will pass and you will find out what seemed like an expensive payment ten years ago is very manageable now. Don't rent; don't refinance; buy and pay off a home so you can become stress free. It's a much better way to live. The future will come so ride the wave.

Thinking about the dollar amounts from today against yesteryear, I came to a funny but startling piece of information in regards to marijuana. Back in the day when I made three dollars an hour an ounce of good Columbian at thirty dollars would figure to be ten times my hourly for one ounce of good pot. When I made thirty-five bucks and hour at retirement a good ounce of meds was $350 per ounce; wouldn't you know. Ten times my hourly wage; who would've thunk. It's funny I don't remember the thirty dollars an ounce to be as dramatic a price as I thought 350 dollars an ounce was. Hmmmm. It was the same percentage in salary.

Anyway, after I decided to retire is when I was about as low as I had ever been. I always looked forward to retirement and anticipated how much fun it was going to be; Not! I was living in a world where a twenty minute nap was king and watching the all night movies was an all too common occurrence. This is about the time Nameless slipped that life changing doobie into my breast pocket. For months it sat in the box while I was asking the same questions my friends asked; "Is this medicine going to help me. I came to find the answer was quite simple; Yes!!!

I don't want anybody to forget what helps me may not be good for you. How something reacts to me may well react in an opposite way for you. Not only that, I can only talk about sleep and how ganja turns off the buzzing so I can find welcome rest. Any other of the dozen maladies marijuana is supposed to relieve is unknown to me so I just can't tell you.

I once receive a prescription from the doctor for codeine to relieve a hacking cough. He told me to watch out and don't drive because it will make me drowsy to the point of falling asleep; wrong! That stuff hit me like a supercharged upper. I had more energy than I knew what to do with so it was obvious it was just the opposite of what the norm is. Coffee is another example. Being my favorite beverage by far, I can drink gallons of it. I use to be able to have a cup of coffee at eight o'clock at night and be sound asleep at ten. The caffeine doesn't seem to bother me in that way. If, however, I have a regular Pepsi or Coke the mixture of caffeine and sugar will assure I wouldn't close my eyes before two A.M. If I have one of those energy drinks I will pull an all night'er if I want to or not. It's strange how a person can react differently from one thing or a mixture of two things. Cannabis is right along these lines. One strain may relax you while it's very uplifting to the next guy. However, speaking about what I know; if sleep is your problem there are more than one strain of Indica that should send you off to meet the Sandman. If you're up dancing and wide eyed after tasting Mrs. Indica then you're a much better man than me. She will send me to dreamland nineteen out of twenty times.

No, nothing works perfectly every time and that includes cannabis. Even though I can rely on it most of the time, there's still some nights that aren't my friend. You don't know how happy I am when I say those night are no longer every night; now it's more like one or two nights a month. But when those nights come it's usually due to a mental anxiety rather than the numb and buzzing arms. If something is in there chewing away at the back of my mind it usually circumvents not only sleep, but peace of mind as well. Grandma used to always tell me you could never relax if something is bothering you; so correct your problems before your go to bed at night. Back then I was a kid without any concept of problems that would keep me from sleeping so, of course, I didn't have a clue to what she was talking about. Now that I think about it she may have been talking about a pissed of spouse instead of outside problems. Back then I would have really not known what she was talking about. Why would problems keep you from fooling around?

Sometimes, not all the time, mind you; but sometimes ganja can work for you even on those rare sleepless nights. After a couple of pulls on the vaporizer between three and four in the morning you will start to relax even if your mind doesn't want to sleep. This is where you can let the herb do its thing by reversing the normal. Remember the guy saying, "You have to pimp the meds, you can't let the meds pimp you?" Here is a time you want the meds to pimp you. You want your thought to flow as free and uninhibited as you can let them; believe me, ganja will let them. As I said, sometimes the free and flowing thoughts will work for you by identifying your anxiety or maybe even finding a solution that was living right below the surface and only visible by a fee flowing thought. When you find the answer your want for sleep will be immediate and you'll be eager to curl back up in bed. On those nights you have a double appreciation for the medication.

So as you can see, or as I tried to explain, medical cannabis has been very beneficial to me in several ways. I don't want anyone to think I'm putting marijuana into the same category as the cure for polio, yellow fever, small pox and penicillin; because I'm not. I'm saying, for me, it opened the door to restful and peaceful sleep; not some nights but most of the nights. Not being sleep weary has benefited my life more than words can explain. Not only has it helped me physically and mentally, it has also given me a very demanding hobby that I can enjoy daily. Between my vegetable garden and the med garden I have the serenity and wonderment of something to fill my days with not to mention watching the earth give up its bountiful harvest. On both counts the consumption is enjoyed and appreciated.

By being your own supplier you not only know what strain you're getting and how it was grown, but as a farmer you can experiment with unknown ways trying to find the better mousetrap. I'm experimenting with a system that seems to be working pretty good for me. Early on I realized the importance of a good cure. Honest to God this will make or break your harvest so treat this step with respect. I found in the cool, slow drying winter the same strains tasted better, smoked smoother and had better potency. The pros say the best drying and curing is around 68 degrees Fahrenheit and I'm not going to be the one arguing with them. Since I live in So Cal my house is ambient most of the time. The winter cool will be in the 50's and a few nights may go all the way down to the forties. The summer day's heat will play in the 80's and 90's with not much more than a week a year breaking the century mark. I'm like a lot of my marijuana strains. I love it in the seventies; I'm happy in the eighties; I begin to wilt in the nineties and I'm truly miserable in the hundreds. Since I dry and cure in a back bedroom shut off from the living area the ambient room could reach temps from the low forties to a hundred and ten; not at all optimal for curing.

I had to find a better way to keep a constant temp for curing. Of course the Frigidaire is too cold for curing. Your weed would turn like limp and slimy celery left in the produce drawer about a month too long. So I tried a system I've heard nobody else talk about. Since the floral bouquets and various flavors are somewhat akin to wine I thought a wine chest might do the trick in regards to a constant temperature. I found a 28 bottle chest with wooden shelves at Home Depot on sale for a buck and a half. This particular model allows you to set the temp from a high of 72 degrees all the way down to a much colder than I need 39. I made a quick stop at the fabric store to purchase a very large nylon mesh; similar as those used in hanging flower dryers. I took a gun and hot glued the mesh very tightly across the wooden shelves so the buds would have air circulating all around them. The glass door was covered with a NASCAR poster cut to the very edge to keep all light away. In the middle there was a cut out revealing a Moni temp and humidity meter so I could know what's going on inside without opening the door.

Now I must admit there are a number of drawbacks with this system. First, when you place a new harvest in a sealed container the humidity skyrockets for the first few days no matter what the temperature. It's almost like curing and drying at the same time. You have to "burp" the chest door several times a day at first but as time goes by the humidity takes longer and longer to raise past my comfort zone. I usually let the humidity get to over 90 percent before I burp the door. The way I do it is just open the door a couple of inches and let a little six inch fan do its thing for two or three minutes. In that time it will bring the moisture down to the ambient 45 percent and evaporate any moisture settling on the buds.

I also use a little packet of silicone gel I got on line from the Rust Store. These little boxes go in the chest and suck moisture out at a very rapid pace. I put one in at 63 grams and took it out two days later at almost 80 grams. When they turn color you just pop them in the microwave or conventional oven to dry them out and they're ready to use again. But beware, after 15 seconds in the microwave the box looks like a steamy Swedish sauna and your kitchen has a beautiful flowery scent; so I dry them at bedtime when I'm not expecting guests. Be sure to get the type WITHOUT cobalt chloride; that crap shouldn't be next to what we consume.

Remember, at sixty-eight degrees it can take up the better part of two weeks in the bud chest before the harvest is ready for the jar; plan another week for curing. This particular chest has a nice feature of having room at the bottom for several curing jars. The shelves of nylon mesh cover almost six square feet so a pretty good size plant has plenty of room for buds with no need to crowd. If you plan your harvest for one plant per month you'll have plenty of time to rotate crops.

Another problem with this system is this is a wine chest cooler; it has no heater. In the summer when the ambient temp might be 80 degrees in the back room the little chest has no problem keeping the buds at a constant 68 degrees. The winter is a different story. The temp can really drop in the back bedroom and, unless you have time to burn, it will take months for ganja to dry in fifty degree temps. I know what you're thinking; just open the back room to the heat of the house. Now, I wouldn't mind doing that except for one small detail. The fruity smell is so thick you could grab a handful, put it in your pocket, take a trip to the grocery store and smell up the whole damn place; that's how extremely fragrant drying bud is. I have to keep the door closed tight or every neighbor on the block will know exactly what I'm doing.

So in the warm weather the wine cabinet works just fine but I had to find a way for a constant cure in the winter. It was a pretty simple remedy. I took one of those clone and seedling warming mats and hung it on the inside of the chest door; perfect. Now the system works in any weather so bring on the harvest. It's not a perfect 68 without a lot of inspections but the time spent will pay off in the quality of meds. Someday I may engineer a system with exhaust fans, tiny electric heaters and humidity meters all hooked up to a control board for hands free curing; on second thought curing should probably always be hands on.

I imagine you can tell there is not too much about ganja that troubles me. Actually, nothing troubles me personally; what troubles me is how outside entities look upon me as a person. I'm sure this is the main reason why up till now I've kept it very personal. I also medicate for medicinal reasons only. To this point I have never used socially with friends or even acquaintances. I'm not sure I would even feel comfortable in an environment like that. Normally I don't medicate during the day unless the night before was an enemy and I need a two hour nap for restitution. I found when you medicate during the day you better have your list of to do's caught up or you may find yourself behind on your chores. Some strains have a way of reorganizing your priorities, which may not bother you at the time, but may force you to put the pedal to the metal when you find you put yourself behind schedule.

Medicating during the day has other problems as far as I'm concerned. I know many people where this doesn't bother them a bit; but it sure bothers me. I really don't like to be around people just after I've medicated; especially the ones I love. Medicating during the day will always lead to somebody dropping by unexpectedly. I don't know why it always happens, but I can usually bet money on it and win. I really feel uncomfortable if the grandkids happen to come over unexpectedly; which has happened once and once was ten times too many. There is no high on earth better than the high two beautiful little faces can give you and I hate anything to muddle the natural. No matter how bad I'm feeling two little voices and a pair of beautiful smiles is more than enough to make Papa's world a very wonderful place.

So, you're about up with me in my walk into medical marijuana. If you've been thinking about taking the walk there are many things to think about before taking the first step:

1) Know yourself. Can you pimp the meds or will the meds pimp you.
2) If you need the herb on a daily basis can you afford the expense to the family budget?
3) If you can't afford the price do you have the ware-with-all to grow your own?

4) If you grow your own can you keep
security secrets? This has to be thought
about very carefully.
5) Are you willing to put in the time and
effort required for quality products?
6) If you're working, does your company
have a random drug testing policy?

These are very important questions and you
should be truthful in your answers. I'm closer to
the view by using this med on a regular basis a
person should truly be up against the wall with no
other way out. But, who am I to say a casual use is
taboo. I'm just not sure a run to the med box every
time you feel a little stress is the right way to use
ganja; just as I don't think a run to the Johnnie
Walker bottle when stressed is any better. Actually,
I think I would rather have the former than the later.

I guess it all comes down to what's the best
path for each individual. Marijuana is probably just
like everything else we consume; it can be used and
it can be abused. I believe it's the user who is
responsible for which path is taken. I didn't want
this writing to say what's best for the reader; I
wanted them to know what's best for me and what I
viewed and experienced on my personal walk. I
don't want people to assume cannabis will help
everyone with their every ill, but on the other hand,

there just may be millions of people marijuana could help if it weren't so belittled by half the society. For me ganja took a man form his whit's end and gave me back the ability to look forward to tomorrow. I'm willing to bet if you don't understand this, then you should thank your God in Heaven your back has never been up against the wall. Not being able to look forward to tomorrow is no place a human being ever wants to be.

So, that's my story and I'm sticking to it. I'm not saying medical marijuana is right or wrong; I'm just saying it has allowed me to look forward to tomorrow. In comparison with not being able to see anything good in the future, now tomorrow is just a day away; and it looks really good from here.

If you're thinking about taking the walk you have many things to think about and to consider. I wish your clear thought in choosing which path you take. I hope your trail is smooth and level and the cold wind is always at your back. Drop me an email and let me know what you think.

With very best regards and good luck to you,

Jeremiah Kush

onemanswalk@gmail.com

www.ingramcontent.com/pod-product-compliance
Lightning Source LLC
Chambersburg PA
CBHW030006190526
45157CB00014B/448